BY
ERNEST D.
SWERSKY,
M.D.

# Outwitting

# Mother Nature

## Why And How To Use Diet Pills

**OUTWITTING MOTHER NATURE**
Why And How To Use Diet Pills

Copyright © 1997 by Ernest D. Swersky, M.D.

ISBN 0-9656544-0-0

Published by:
Ernest D. Swersky, M.D.

Printed by:
Personal Profiles Publishing Co.
Dallas, Texas

Printed in the United States of America
First Printing

All rights reserved. No part of this publication may be reproduced, stored in a retrieval system, or transmitted in any form by any means, electronic, mechanical, photocopy, recording, or otherwise, without prior written permission from the publisher, with the exception of short excerpts used with acknowledgment of publisher.

# Dedication

*This book is dedicated to that group of people,
my patients, who have given me the greatest gift
one person can give to another:
trust.*

# Acknowledgments

*I would like to acknowledge the support of my wife Paula and my son Aaron in the writing of this book. I would like to particularly acknowledge the help of my son David, who has helped keep me on track and who has believed in this project from the beginning.*

*I would also like to thank Beverly Forté for her advice. I am particularly indebted to David Stanley, without whose help this book could not have happened.*

# Table of Contents

| | |
|---|---|
| Introduction | 1 |
| 1: How I Became A Weight Loss "Expert" | 7 |

## Part I: Why We're Overweight

| | |
|---|---|
| 2: Our Conflict With Mother Nature | 19 |

## Part II: What We've Done About It Before

| | |
|---|---|
| 3: How Our Attitudes Have Changed | 35 |
| 4: The Amphetamine Disaster | 41 |
| 5: The Weight Loss Industry | 49 |
| 6: The Misuse Of Psychology In Weight Loss | 63 |
| 7: The Misunderstanding Of Exercise In Weight Loss | 69 |

## Part III: What To Do About It

| | |
|---|---|
| 8: How Does All This Apply To You? | 77 |
| 9: An Ethical Weight Loss Program | 85 |
| 10: Evaluation And Examination | 89 |

| | |
|---|---|
| 11: Program Design | 99 |
| 12: Informed Consent | 109 |
| 13: Follow-Up | 115 |
| 14: Giving It Up | 119 |
| | |
| Appendix A: The Appetite Suppressants | 123 |
| Appendix B: Informed Consent Forms | 139 |
| Appendix C: References | 145 |

# Introduction

The fact that you are holding this book in your hands is a testament to the resilience of the human spirit.

If you are like most of us who have fought the weight war, you are once again attempting to find the answer to a chronic problem in your life, overweight. Perhaps you've tried diets only to fail at them, or, even worse, perhaps you've succeeded in losing weight only to have it return with a vengeance as soon as you let down your guard. Of course, no one told you that these diets have been shown in independent studies to have a success rate of lower than 5%. If the promoters of these diets had been honest, you would probably have made a different choice and saved yourself a lot of money and pain.

On the other hand, you may be considering entering the bewildering maze of weight loss for the first time.

As you look at the shelves of diet books in your local book store, supermarket, or magazine store, you may be confused by the conflicting claims made by various authors. Some will tell you that it's the kind of food you eat that's the problem; others will tell you that it's just a matter of mind over body. All of them will present the *answers* in such a way as to make them seem self evident and simple.

The TV ads all make the store front programs seem like the simplest, easiest, most effective, and successful answers to your problem. It's obvious from all the pictures of the smiling faces that they've found the ultimate answer to their overweight problem, and the advertisers are just waiting for you to join the ranks of their satisfied customers.

Not until you try these answers once, and again, and again, will you begin to realize that they don't work for you. Of course, you feel that the failure must be your fault, because it says right there on the cover of the book that so and so is an "expert" in nutrition, or diet, or some other field. Not only is the author an expert, but the first cousin of the garbage man who picks up the trash from some celebrity's house has personally endorsed this program as *The Answer*.

It's also clear from the ads on TV that everyone else who has ever tried the program has succeeded, and you must be the only person in the whole world who has failed to achieve and maintain your goals permanently.

So you lick your wounds and marvel at how weak you are, and punish yourself with the biggest, juiciest, greasiest hamburger in the known universe, *with* large fries and a Coke.

The one minor detail that all of these "experts" seem to have overlooked is the answer to a very simple question: why are we overweight? They all assume that the answer is so simple that the question is unnecessary. Everyone knows that overweight is caused by eating too much, so why bother?

The real question should be: ***why*** do we eat too much?

Are we a nation of gluttons? Doesn't anyone care about weight? Are we all weak? Do we all have some character flaw that makes us lack will power? Or is it just possible that the answer is "none of the above"? Is it possible that all we are doing is what comes naturally in an unnatural environment?

This book is about understanding the failure of diets alone as a means for controlling overweight. It looks at a combination of natural history, human behavior, the human brain, and the market place, and shows the misconceptions, misunderstandings and downright lies that have prevented the effective treatment of overweight for many years. It explains that we become overweight by doing exactly what we're supposed to do, that is, satisfy our hunger, and that we have no choice in the matter by nature's design. In an exclusive interview with Mother Nature, we'll even see why we'll have to outwit her if we're going to solve the problem.

The first chapter tells the story of my rather undistinguished attempts to treat the overweight problem in my patients and how I finally figured out what I had been doing wrong.

In Part I, we'll look at the reasons why such a large proportion of the population of the developed world is overweight. If we follow the simple principle that the vast majority of people behave the way they're supposed to, then the challenge becomes understanding the forces that cause this behavior. The behavior in question is eating too much for our own long-term good. This is where we'll see how our brains are designed so that our human agenda must take second place to the agenda designed into us by Mother Nature.

The second part of this book is a look at the ways we've tried to deal with the problem of overweight in the past. It looks at the efforts that have been made to understand our overeating and the reasons why these efforts have been such a dismal failure. You'll also see the kinds of answers to the problem of overweight that have been tried, and some of the well-intentioned, and not so well-intentioned, methods that have been offered to us from the so called "experts" in the field. You'll also see how ridiculous many of these "answers" are in the face of the facts.

The third part of this book shows you, in great detail, exactly how the problem of overweight can be addressed by an informed consumer. Whether you want to lose just a few pounds, or whether you have been very overweight all of your life, this book will be a blueprint of the safest and most reasonable ways for you to approach your weight problem.

There are some sacrifices you'll have to make if you decide to use this program. You'll have to give up the blame and guilt for being overweight. You'll have to give up the hunger that has always gone with dieting. You'll have to give up the idea of using will power as a means of putting up with the misery of dieting. You'll also have to give up the idea that it's entirely your responsibility to lose weight, and learn to share that responsibility with a doctor who is prepared to help you find a medication that is right for you. Perhaps most importantly, you will also have to give up the idea that treating overweight is a temporary effort, and demand of your doctor that your problem be taken seriously just as if you had diabetes or high blood pressure.

Freedom has a price. In this case the price is changing the way we think about ourselves. The reward for paying that price is the ability to see ourselves as the beautiful, natural people we are as well as the liberation from all of the guilt and blame for being overweight.

# CHAPTER 1

# How I Became A Weight Loss "Expert"

Doctors are not trained to deal with the overweight problem. There are no medical school courses called "Weight Loss 101." Because of this, it's up to the individual doctor to decide whether and how to deal with the problem as a matter of personal preference. The experiences, prejudices, and attitudes of the individual practitioner have, up to now, driven all of his or her decisions about whether and how to treat overweight. Most doctors choose not to deal with the problem once they see how useless the usual answers prove to be.

My education in weight loss began in a round about

way while I was an undergraduate student. There's a rule that says that every undergraduate student must, at least once in his or her college career, get so far behind at exam time that "pulling an all nighter," that is studying all night before an exam, seems like a good idea. It's in the chapter of the rule book called "Really Stupid Things You Must Do Before You Can Graduate." Subsection three of this rule says that you get extra points for taking amphetamines to help you through the night and the exam the next day.

In compliance with this rule, I got seriously behind in one of my chemistry courses and decided to go through the "all nighter" ritual for an afternoon exam the following day. I took my first amphetamine pill at about two in the morning and took one about every four hours until just before the exam at two in the afternoon. I did okay until about six in the evening when the effects began to wear off, and then I took a nose dive.

The depression, irritability, achiness, and general misery lasted for about another four hours. I was going through withdrawal after four doses! I figured I'd take these pills again just as soon as hell freezes over. I needed no convincing that amphetamines were bad news. No wonder they were not allowed to be prescribed for weight loss any more!

My education continued with my medical school training at Dalhousie University in Halifax, Nova Scotia, one of the oldest medical schools in North America. The only time weight loss was ever mentioned in medical school was to warn us about the side effects and addictive potential of the only class of medications then available known to suppress the appetite, the amphetamines. My experience with the amphetamines as an undergraduate made the warning unnecessary.

Dalhousie provided me with a solid background in almost all the areas necessary to be a competent doctor. I say almost because, like most medical educations, there was nothing in my training about nutrition. I learned some of the most minute details about human beings but nothing about the fuel that makes them work — sort of a course in the care and feeding of human beings without the feeding.

My first practice was in the Acadian French town of Shediac, in the Canadian province of New Brunswick. Now, anyone who has ever been to Louisiana can appreciate the fact that Acadians, called Cajuns in the US, are not a particularly skinny group. They have their fair share of seriously overweight people, most of whom, it seemed, wanted to see what the new doctor in town had to offer in the way of the latest advances in weight loss.

The new doctor in town was required to have an answer for everything, so I mumbled something about balanced diets and will power. The good people of Shediac soon realized that I was just as useless in the area of weight loss as all the rest of the doctors in town and stopped bothering to ask me for help in the area.

There were several new appetite suppressants developed in the seventies. Once, in about 1974, a pharmaceutical company's representative came by my office and assured me that his company's new appetite suppressant was safe and effective and had almost no side effects. Since I had begun to expand in the waist department from the consequences of a happily married life, I thought that I'd give one of them a try, purely for the benefit of my patients you understand. My experience with that particular dosage of that particular medication was an uncomfortable one. I had many of the stimulant side effects of appetite suppressants without understanding that these side effects are usually very short-lived and usually wear off after a short time. Because of my ignorance, I immediately branded all appetite suppressants as bad for me and my patients. I also reasoned that since diets didn't work for anybody else I wasn't going to bother with them either.

In 1978 my wife, my two sons, and I moved to Dallas. Once again, as soon as my new patients in Dallas discovered just how "expert" I was at dealing with the problem of overweight, they stopped asking me for any useful answers.

Things went on like this until I ran across a former classmate, Nate, who had moved to Dallas one year after we did and began a practice in ophthalmology. Over the years, he, too, had begun to fight the battle of the bulge, but when I saw him in late 1990 he looked great. He had lost about twenty pounds and couldn't say enough good things about this new diet that had worked so well for him. Nate is an Energizer Bunny kind of guy, and he insisted that I look into trying this new program in my practice. I guess his enthusiasm was infectious, because I actually listened to him. It turned out that Nate was using one of the

new liquid protein diets called Medifast®.
Medifast®, like Optifast® of Oprah fame, is a type of diet known as a Very Low Calorie Diet, or VLCD. These diets allow people to lose weight very quickly, and they were very popular in the late eighties and early nineties. They consisted of about 580 calories a day of concentrated nutrients, vitamins, and minerals, taken in the form of a sort of milk shake. One of the biggest reasons for the success of these diets was that people ate absolutely no food, and, therefore, weren't constantly tempted to cheat — sort of cold turkey without the turkey.

I decided that the only ethical way to offer the Medifast® program was to combine it with a series of lectures, designed to make it perfectly clear to my patients that this was just a gimmick to get the weight off and that the real program was the maintenance phase. I even offered the maintenance part free after my patients reached their goals. None of this regain stuff for my patients!

At first everything went well. Almost everyone lost weight very quickly and almost everyone found the program to be relatively easy. However, it quickly became obvious that as soon as my patients were reintroduced to food they began to regain all of their weight, and disappeared. In a few cases they came back sheepishly for a "refresher," but, in most cases, they just vanished. A couple I'll call Fred and Mary were the last straw.

> Fred and Mary came to my program by word of mouth. Fred weighed 422 pounds, and his wife Mary weighed 240 pounds. These are two of the nicest folks you could ever hope to meet. Fred is a computer systems

engineer, and Mary is a software writer. Their dream was to be "normal" and not to be judged by the world in terms of their weight. They took their protein supplements religiously and even cleared all of the food out of their house. Not only did they attend all of the lectures, but they even went around for a second time.

Fred lost 200 pounds in exactly the time it took Mary to lose 100 pounds, and I almost broke my arm patting myself on the back. Three hundred pounds! Then Mary added to the excitement by getting pregnant. They had been infertile, probably because of the hormonal problems associated with extreme overweight, but now their last obstacle to fulfillment as a couple was gone. We had just finished the food reintroduction and were beginning maintenance when they, too, disappeared.

The next time I saw Mary was after the baby was born. She was well on her way to regaining all of her weight and, she informed me, so was Fred. By this time I had already recognized that this was the rule rather than the exception and had stopped offering the Medifast® program to my patients.

I had failed. No matter how hard I tried, and, more importantly, no matter how hard my patients tried, almost everyone regained their weight as soon as they were reintroduced to food. When it came time for people to exercise their will power, it just didn't work. The whole premise of my program had been that an honest presentation of the process coupled with a clear message about what would be required for long-term success would work. It didn't.

For the next few years I refused to treat weight problems. Whenever they asked, I told my patients that because I didn't know how to help them keep the weight off, I wasn't going to put them through the misery, and risks, of taking it off. I told my patients that medical science just didn't have the answer to the overweight problem, and, until the answer was discovered, I had nothing to offer them.

My attitude was pretty much unchanged until early summer of 1995 when I started hearing about "phen fen." Several patients asked me my opinion about this new weight loss idea. When I finally figured out that this was a combination of two of the newer weight loss medications initially introduced in the seventies, my immediate response was, to be charitable, less than enthusiastic. This was the dumbest idea I had ever heard of. As if one of these pills wasn't dangerous enough, now we'll combine two of them and really mess some people up! Of all the stupid ideas, this one really took the cake.

Patients kept asking about this phen fen stuff until I became alarmed about the situation and decided to research it for myself. I wanted to warn them about the real dangers of this hare-brained idea from an authoritative point of view. Other people might try this new fad, but at least my patients would be educated as to its dangers. I called my hospital library and had them pull all the information they could get their hands on about *phen*termine and *fen*fluramine. A couple of days later, I picked up the studies and set about arming myself against this new threat to my patients' health.

Many of the studies were on one of the medications alone or mentioned both in passing, and a lot of them mentioned a study[1] done at the University of Syracuse

School of Medicine and Dentistry by a doctor named Weintraub. Finally I came to the Weintraub study itself. Aha! Paydirt. Now let's see what kind of foolishness we're dealing with here.

Hmm, seems well designed. Hmm, well written from a scientific point of view. Hmm, analysis of the data seems well done. Let's see now, 40% success rate — wow! But what about the risks of this new combination of medications? Hmm, okay but the side effects were. . . hmm, not bad. I'll bet the addiction problem bit them in the you know where. . . no addiction, interesting.

Finally, the fly in the ointment, the smoking gun, the proof of the crime! It says right here that even after four years, as soon as people stopped the medications they put all of their weight right back on! I knew this wouldn't work. I knew it was too good to be true. You'd have to keep people on this stuff forever for it to solve their overweight problem, and everyone knows you can't do that. . . Hmm, I take my blood pressure medication every day — It's safe except for a few minor side effects in some patients. . . hmmm.

The study showed that phen fen produced effective weight loss about 40% of the time, which is a lot better than the less than 5% effectiveness of the fad diets. It also showed that phen fen was well tolerated. All of the observed side effects went away when the medication was stopped, and none were dangerous. It was not addictive, and worked as long as it was used. Then, as they say, the penny dropped.

The importance of the research is not that phen fen works, although that is an important finding. The importance is in the fact that the people in the program were unable to maintain their weight loss without the medication.

***It's not about the medication.* This phen fen stuff is not what this research is all about. *It's about giving people control over hunger!***

The more I thought about it the more it made sense. Phen fen works because it stops ***hunger.***

# Hunger is the enemy!

Armed with new enthusiasm, I decided to offer my patients phentermine and fenfluramine, among other appetite suppressants, as a part of my practice. My experience has been very rewarding. I'm now able to approach the problem of overweight in a way that offers the best chance of success available at the present time. I'm able to approach the treatment of this condition from the same angle that I approach any other major risk factor, that is, safely and permanently. I'm also able to do so in the atmosphere of scientific validity on which I've always tried to base my practice.

As I was promoting the idea to my patients, I ended up answering a lot of questions in my own mind about why appetite suppression is an important key to permanent weight loss. I also answered many of the questions that had plagued me about the failure of the Medifast® program. Some of these questions are:

- Why do people become overweight in the first place?
- Why can't people follow a "sensible" diet?
- Why doesn't will power work?
- Why do people regain their weight once they've gone through all the trouble to lose it in the first place?

Let's begin to look at the problem of overweight by looking at the subject of the problem: humans.

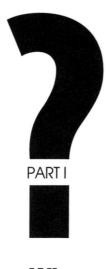

# Why We're Overweight

# CHAPTER 2

# Our Conflict With Mother Nature

**N**ature is what we call the set of rules that governs how the planet works. Some of us call it by religious names, some of us call it by scientific names; all of us are trying to define it in our own terms. This set of rules is not under our control. We can't repeal the law of gravity, and we can't change the wave lengths of light to which our eyes respond. We can't change the way that genetic information is passed on from one generation to another, nor can we change the nature of that genetic information. We also can't control the basic survival instincts, like hunger, that have been programmed into us by nature.

What we can do is use our ability to think. With this ability we can understand the difference between the ways nature defines us and the ways we want to be defined. Another way of saying this is that we can understand the conflict between nature's agenda for us and our own agenda for ourselves.

## Mother Nature's Agenda – Survival

Nature has devised a way for each life form to get the necessary supply of energy, or food, for its survival in one way or another. In the case of a life form such as a fern, this energy comes directly from the sun through the fern's leaves. In the case of more complicated life forms like humans, this energy is released by the breakdown of what we call food.

Food is the fuel of life. When the supply of fuel stops, so does life. This is a non-negotiable requirement of survival as shown by the fate of the dinosaurs. After millions of years, the dinosaurs' food supply suddenly dried up. Mother Nature must have been really annoyed when that asteroid hit. All that effort down the drain, but, them's the rules; no second chances or time outs. "Can't feed yerself? Yer outta here!"

That's a tough rule to live by if you happen to be a life form, because one of the other rules of the game is that you live in a constant state of fear about the supply of food. If Mother Nature gets distracted, say, building fjords on the coast of Norway and forgets to make it rain in your neck of the woods, you'd better be able to hold out until she gets back to you. If you forget to put a little something away for a snack when you need it, usually in the form of some stored fat, don't expect any sympathy from her. If you're gonna wimp out just because of a little drought, then give Ma Nature's regards to the dinosaurs.

The lesson to be learned from these observations is an important step in understanding the role of hunger in the development of humanity.

**The constant need for food in an atmosphere of nutritional insecurity is one of the forces which dictate the nature of all life on the planet, including Man.**

Food and its acquisition are central to our basic biological natures. There is absolutely nothing optional about eating. It's a basic survival behavior. Mother Nature has equipped us for survival with a special control system in our brain. This control system is designed to send us a constant barrage of signals, and these signals are sent to remind us to protect ourselves against our nutritional insecurity. These signals are called *hunger*. When we look at the control system that governs hunger, we can see how Mother Nature prioritized this system and why we can't control the signals it sends us.

### *How the Brain Controls Hunger*

The forebrain, those enormous cerebral hemispheres, is where our conscious minds live. This is the part of the brain that's responsible for abilities such as reasoning and self awareness. It's the part of the brain in which our personalities live and from which we reach out to the world and try to make it conform to our wishes. This is the level at which our human agenda arises.

The midbrain is where the control of our instinctive behavior is located. These behaviors are controlled by preprogrammed instructions, and these instructions are, for the most part, completely invisible to our conscious minds. In other words, the midbrain defines the environment in which our minds, contained in our forebrains, live. The midbrain is the area where nature's agenda for us is expressed.

One of the areas of the midbrain is called the thalamus. Under this area is located one of the most important control centers of the brain called the hypothalamus. Some of the things the hypothalamus controls are the drive to reproduce, the level of our metabolism, the need for sleep, and the level of our hunger. It's the control of hunger that we're interested in here.

The expression of hunger is exactly the same in a four hundred pound man as it is in a one hundred pound woman. The only difference is one of degree. The differences in the levels of these drives from person to person are determined by our genes and these genes are expressed by controls which are located in the hypothalamus. Here's how it works.

The hypothalamus is wired directly into the "pleasure center" of the brain and communicates its messages to the pleasure center through the release of a neurotransmitter. A neurotransmitter is a chemical messenger that nerve cells use to send each other signals. The particular neurotransmitter used by the hypothalamus to communicate with the pleasure center of the brain is called serotonin.

When we do the things that nature wants us to do, we get a *yum* message from the release of serotonin to the pleasure center, and when we do something that endangers us, we get an *ugh* message by getting some serotonin taken away. Rule number one in nature's manual on *How To Be a Life Form* is "Go for the *yums*, avoid the *ughs.*" Remember, this is not conscious; it's automatic. We're not aware of these drives; we just live by them.

Research has shown that if you hook a rat up to a *yum* stimulator implanted directly into its brain, it will press the *yum* button until it dies of starvation with a smile on its little face. You can witness the same phenomenon in humans in any crack house in the country. Narcotics stimulate the release of serotonin in the human pleasure center. When a person craves this stimulation through the use of a drug we call this an addiction.

> **When the same person craves this stimulation through the intake of food we call this <u>hunger</u>.**

That's why you don't see a lot of chubby addicts. They've got a virtual *yum* button implanted directly into their brains that they push by using drugs. Why should they bother with the relatively weak *yum* provided by food when they can get an enormous **YUM** from crack cocaine?

What the addict has done is to find a substance which satisfies the pleasure center of the brain in exactly the same way that food does but to an abnormal extent. The point is:

## Hunger is a drive and not just a sensation.

"So what's this guy saying, that we're all addicted to food?" In effect, yes, just like we're all "addicted" to the other things necessary for the survival of the species like oxygen, sleep, and reproductive behavior, known as sex. Nature uses the reward of serotonin to the pleasure center as a way to make us behave in ways guaranteed to ensure our survival — sort of a pat on the head for good behavior. Nature's goal for all of our behaviors is survival.

An *ugh* is the equivalent of a rap on the nose with a newspaper. It's known as an aversive stimulant, and it happens when we get some serotonin taken away from our pleasure centers. Some of the common *ughs* are things like fear, lack of stimulation known as boredom, anxiety, pain, and, you guessed it — hunger.

Of course, we would like to think we're beyond all that outmoded instinctive stuff. After all, we have this marvelous new invention called the cerebral hemispheres, these large, fancy, convoluted gizmos that make up by far the largest part of our brains. This is where we've developed our self awareness, along with the idea that we can control nature.

**What we've been doing to control our hunger in the past is to try to use these cerebral hemispheres to out-vote the instinctive parts of our brain. We've tried to impose our conscious agendas on our unconscious minds.**

The problem with this is that no matter how hard we try, we can't convince our hypothalamus to release the serotonin to turn the *ugh* of hunger into the *yum* we crave unless we eat enough food to do it. That's why will power must fail. The *will* is not in the same place as the *power*.

It seems that nature is too smart to give us upstarts the final word about the really important survival issues. She has retained a veto which can be wielded by the hypothalamus in case we try to do something really stupid like, say, get thin.

> "Can you imagine that? I, Mother Nature, go through all the trouble to make you hungry so that you don't starve, I get you through the ice ages, I get you through wars, I develop those fancy cerebral hemispheres for you to play with, and what thanks do I get? The first chance you get you want to throw it all away by being thin. Haven't I taught you anything? It's a jungle out there. Think of all those extinct species."

> "Aw Ma, it's not like that any more. You just don't understand. All that survival stuff is, like, out dated. It's not cool to be chubby Ma. Thin is In."

> "Don't you talk back to your mother, young human. I'm the boss in this house and what I say goes. You can diet, you can exercise, you can whine all you want, but I'll have the last word. You will listen to your hypothalamus and do what it tells you. It's much older and smarter than you are. Now go get a little snack and you'll feel better."

Who's right? They both are. They just have different agendas. Who wins? Mother Nature, of course. She's stacked the deck by putting the hypothalamus in control. She has provided us with the means to survive the realities of the natural environment. Her agenda, survival, is responsible for us making it this far.

The human agenda is different, for reasons which make perfect sense to us, but which are, by definition, in conflict with our design. Our agenda has gone beyond our survival as a species to the health and well being of the individual.

## The Human Agenda – Quality of Life

At first we followed the rules. We took what nature gave us when she chose to be generous and did the best we could in the hard times. But over the millennia, we used the brains Mother Nature gave us to develop tools that allowed us to change the environment rather than accept things as they were. We used those tools to help in the gathering and preparation of food, and, as we developed further understanding of how our environments worked, we developed better tools and methods to help us increase our food supply.

Until around the end of the last century, much of the population of this nation still suffered nutritional insecurity. A huge proportion of the American people continued to work on the land, some providing enough food only for their own families, some not even that. Around the turn of the century things began to change.

Advances in land use, seed quality, farm machinery, animal husbandry, and distribution began to create surpluses of food. In prior systems these surpluses belonged to the land owners who could use them to line their own pockets, but, in the system of American democracy, the producer was free to offer these surpluses, for a fair price, to the population at large. This has resulted in an unprecedented level of food availability.

In this country, we spend the smallest proportion of our income on food of any people on earth. In every town there are restaurants that provide cheap, nutritious food at a low price. Even when we do prepare our own food, we have an incredible variety of cheap foods available, many of them already partly ready to eat. The rarest delicacies of fifty years ago are commonplace today.

It should come as no surprise that the hypothalamus hasn't gotten the news yet. As far as it is concerned, it's business as usual with famine lurking around the next corner. It goes about its job of making us hungry so that we eat as if we were still hunting and gathering and foraging for our sustenance like we were doing yesterday.

In a matter of one century, our relationship to food has undergone a complete about-face while our hypothalamus hasn't changed. As a result, we've progressed from the natural condition of not having enough food to the new problems associated with an unlimited supply. These are the problems of overnutrition.

Now that we are living longer, partly because of the abundance of food, that very abundance is causing some of the worst diseases we have to face in old age. The majority of these diseases are directly caused by being overweight. We've outsmarted our own natures where nutrition is concerned.

The success of the American system has allowed us a large number of luxuries. One of the most important of these is the development of an entire new agenda for our lives. We are no longer content with surviving long enough to reproduce and raise a family. Our new goal is to survive to a leisure age, beyond the responsibilities of parenting, and even beyond the responsibilities of earning a living. We want to retire and be well enough, and well off enough, to reap the rewards of our labors. The American dream is no longer "making it," but "enjoying it." Unfortunately, that dream brings us, once again, head-to-head with nature.

Nature is not a democrat; she designs species, not individuals. Success, as far as she's concerned, is survival to successful reproduction. Anything else is totally unnecessary.

"Uh, Ma Nature, can we talk?"

"Yes dear, what is it?"

"Well, it looks like we've got this nutrition thing pretty well under control."

"Yes, and I'm proud of you. You're the first ones to figure out how to look after yourselves. It's nice to be able to go off and do something without having to worry about finding you've all starved to death when I come back."

"Yeah, we're kind of glad about that too, but we've been thinking, like you taught us to do, and we'd like to ask you a favor."

"What is it?"

"Well, you know how the rules say - eat, reproduce, and get out of the way? Well, we wondered if we could sort of hang around after we're finished reproducing?"

"I guess so. Now run off and get a snack and let me finish this planet."

"Well, you see, that's just the problem. All this snacking with all of this food is causing us to have health problems and die at an early age, so could you turn off the hypothalamus so we could live longer?"

"Right, you want me to redesign the whole system just because you've figured out how to feed yourselves. If you're so smart, figure it out for yourselves. Now run along and play with that fancy brain I gave you."

We've already "figured out" other problems like this one. The control of stage fright is a perfect example.

Some people suffer from crippling physical symptoms when they have to speak in front of an audience. Their mouths get as dry as powder, their hearts race, they tremble, and they feel like they can't breathe normally. We used to think of this as a psychological problem and people spent years in therapy trying to overcome these symptoms. We now know that these symptoms are directly caused by the sudden release of a flood of adrenaline into their blood streams in response to fear. If these people take a medication called propranolol, known as Inderal®, before this starts, it just doesn't happen. The medication blocks the effect of adrenaline on the body. The adrenaline is still produced. It just doesn't cause all of the symptoms. We've got that problem figured out.

Another example of our use of the ol' brain is how we deal with high blood pressure. Some of the medications we use act in the central nervous system to block the messages that cause the blood pressure to rise. The messages still get sent, but they don't get through. We've pretty well figured that one out as well.

The bottom line is that if Ma Nature won't redesign the hypothalamus for us, it's up to us to figure out how to manage it in such a way so that we can live by our own agendas. It so happens that this has already been done. The appetite suppressants actually prevent the hunger signals from being sent to the brain. They block the *ugh* signal from the hypothalamus. Here's what we've figured out about overweight:

- Hunger is not just a sensation. It's a drive that's programmed into our unconscious minds as a basic survival mechanism.

- The hunger mechanism is not responsive to human control. The level of the brain in which it lives is a primitive level which takes precedence over our conscious minds.

- It is impossible for the human animal to go hungry for extended periods of time if there is an alternative. We are designed to acquire energy, not only for our immediate needs, but in case of need in the future.

- The level of hunger in any given individual is a function of the genetic programming of the hypothalamus, and there is no way to reprogram it once we are conceived.

- It is up to us to devise ways to control this system after the fact. Wishing things were different won't get us to our goals. Will power won't do it either.

These are the facts about ourselves that we have to work with if we're ever going to find a solution to the overweight problem. We've got to find a way to free ourselves from the limitations of our natural design.

Of course, things are never simple when it comes to us humans. In our attempts to deal with the problem of overweight, we've led ourselves down some dead end paths and fallen over a few cliffs. Those past failures still affect the ways we use to lose weight. If we don't want to relive history we're going to have to learn from it.

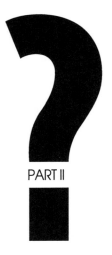

PART II

# What
# We've Done About It Before

# CHAPTER 3
# How Our Attitudes Have Changed

As the food supply increased at the turn of this century, the general populace began to put on weight. At first, this may have been thought to be a positive thing. After all, just a few years ago thin meant either sick or poor. If we look at post cards, pictures, publications, and bathing beauties from that era, we see men who look pretty average, that is, not models, and women who look downright overweight. These illustrations are signs of their times. *Plumpness* was a positive sign of beauty. These women's shapes were defined by the layer of adipose tissue (fat) covering the underlying muscle. Muscularity was seen as unattractive, and the more her muscles showed through, the less attractive the woman was judged to be.

After the First World War in the teens and twenties, the perception of beauty changed dramatically. With the development of the economic boom, food was less and less a problem. Now, all of the fashion illustrations were of tall, lanky women. It became *in to be thin*. Fred Astaire was the model of thinness, and he was a caricature of it. The specter of hunger was fading from the minds of the American public.

The economic crash of 1929 was the beginning of the end for this thinness craze. With so many people destitute, the supply of food became not only an individual concern but a national concern as well. Entire populations were living on the edge of subsistence, and, once again, the specter of hunger ruled people's imaginations. If we look at the movies of this era, we can judge the attitude towards weight by how the *beautiful* woman looked. *Plumpness* was back in. Mae West was the ideal of femininity, and she was, to be generous, plump. Thinness was a luxury people couldn't afford.

After the Second World War, economic growth and prosperity returned. Now the ideals of beauty were the *superwomen* with all of their curves exaggerated but still covered and defined by a layer of fat. Marilyn Monroe was the ideal of the fifties and, as I have heard from a number of women of varying sizes, none of them small, Marilyn was *not* thin.

Jump ahead a few decades and look at the eighties and nineties. For the most part, the availability of cheap, nutritious food is only a few minutes away. We've lived with prosperity long enough that the fear of hunger has faded, and we now judge beauty in terms of underlying muscle and bone structure covered by a very thin layer of fat. The problem with this model is that it has no relationship to the amount of fat carried by the average person. It is once again *in to be thin*, and the level of thinness that's *in* is not natural. This book would be an appeal to the American public to accept their natural weight as beautiful if it were not for the health risks of being overweight that were identified by medical studies.

**Overweight is no longer merely
a cosmetic problem.
It's a major health problem as well.**

## *Health Risks*

The first study to raise a fuss about the health risks of overweight was the Framingham Study[3] done in the late fifties and early sixties in Framingham, Massachusetts, by researchers from Harvard University. This was the important study that linked smoking to cancer and heart disease. It also linked high cholesterol and high blood pressure to heart disease and showed overweight to be a risk factor in all of these diseases as well. In studies on the causes of chronic diseases, the weight of the individual appeared consistently as a positive risk for the disease. Over the next fifteen to twenty years, the evidence became overwhelming.

**Overweight is one of — if not the greatest —
treatable risk factor for disease in the US**

The risks of overweight include: hypertension,[4] cardiovascular disease,[5] stroke,[6] gall stones,[7] diabetes,[8] pulmonary disease,[9] gout,[10] and, cancers of the breast,[11] uterus,[12] endometrium,[13] prostate,[14] colon and rectum,[15] and testicle.[16] Overweight also causes increased risk in surgical patients[17] and in pregnancy.[18]

With the possible exception of cigarette smoking, there is no other single risk factor that is associated with so much human suffering. This list doesn't even cover the issues of self esteem and prejudice in the home, in the workplace, in social situations, and in the hearts of people who struggle with the problem of overweight.

One of the first consequences of these medical findings was to legitimize the quest for thinness. Until quite recently, weight loss has been seen as only a cosmetic issue by many doctors as well as the governmental agencies associated with public health. As a cosmetic issue, it was often dismissed as frivolous and not serious enough to justify the risk of using medications.

It has been estimated that one third of the American public is now overweight.[19] As the medical community realized the prevalence and the seriousness of the problem and as the public health agencies realized the human and economic cost of overweight, those attitudes have undergone a dramatic change.

### *Chronic Health Problem*

It is now accepted that the treatment for overweight needs to be approached in exactly the way we look at the treatment for high blood pressure, diabetes, heart disease, or any other chronic health problem. We need to treat this problem, within the bounds of acceptable risk, scientifically and permanently. Overweight also needs to be seen from the perspective of a permanent biological problem which deserves serious medical intervention. It is time for the medical community and the public to take the management of the problem away from the weight loss gurus and to rely on fact instead of fiction.

So, what's the problem? We know diets don't work, but we still view the only alternative, the appetite suppressants, with suspicion. What's the difference between using medication to treat one cause of heart disease, high blood pressure, and to treat another cause, overweight? Why should one be seen as the standard of good care and the other be viewed with suspicion and fear? The answer lies in the experience with the amphetamine disaster in the 1930s.

CHAPTER 4

# The Amphetamine Disaster

There are some very good reasons why people are wary of taking a medication to treat overweight. Medications can cause side effects, and they're not 100% effective, but the most common reasons people give for their hesitancy are the product of misinformation. The basis for this misinformation lies in the disastrous history of the use of amphetamines. These were the first medications discovered to reduce the *demand* for food by suppressing the appetite. Up to that point, all attempts to lose weight had been restricted to reducing only the *supply* of food with the usual consequences, failure.

## *The Amphetamines of the Thirties*

When amphetamines were discovered in the thirties, we thought that the final answer to the overweight problem had been found! As soon as you turned off the *demand* for food in the brain, weight loss became a snap.

People flocked to doctor's offices to get their hands on this great new miracle pill. Forget about all those failed diets. This was the answer. Besides, not only did almost everyone lose weight quickly and effortlessly, they felt great as well. They had lots of energy and a sense of well being. "Boy, if I'd known how great it felt to be thin I would have done this years ago." There was certainly no problem getting people to take the pills on a regular schedule. As a matter of fact, people never wanted to stop them.

> "Ladies and gentlemen of the worshipping public. I, Doctor of the Thirties, come here to accept this award for the discovery of the amphetamines. Because we haven't yet invented antibiotics and because we are still in the beginning stages of learning to treat most diseases, it is gratifying to know that we have at least one solution that really works."
>
> "Pssst."
>
> "I'm sure as we continue to look for . . ."
>
> "Pssst."
>
> "Go away, can't you see I'm giving a speech? Ahem. Where was I . . . ?"

"Psssssst."

"What is it?"

"Well doc, there seems to be a little problem with those amphetamines. It appears that they cause a dangerous increase in blood pressure in some people, and they've been associated with lots of deaths from heart attacks and strokes."

"Er, ah."

"Oh yeah, they're fiercely addicting, they also cause severe personality changes, and sometimes they cause paranoia. Whatsamatter, doc? You don't look very well."

"Well, I'd have to see the studies, and, and er . . ."

"Don't worry yerself about it, doc. The state and federal agencies have already taken them off the shelves, so you won't have to prescribe them anymore."

"What am I supposed to do with all of my patients who were taking this stuff? You mean to tell me that they're all *addicted*? We haven't even invented the tranquilizers yet. What am I supposed to do with them?"

"Go into the treatment of addiction as a career change?"

"Get out of here and let me finish making a fool of myself in front of all these people."

Picture yourself back in the thirties. You live in the middle of the Great Depression, but you're one of the lucky ones with lots to eat. You're overweight, and you've been dieting on and off for years, and then you think they've finally come up with *the* answer — the amphetamines.

After about a year of taking these new diet pills, you're doing great! For some reason, you're taking more than when you started to get the same result, but, hey, results count. You're slim and trim, and you've got enough energy to lick your weight in wildcats. You may be irritable, but it's all your boss' fault anyway. It's time for a refill, so you trot down to your local drug store. The pharmacist informs you that those pills you've been taking have been taken off the market. So you call your doctor for an alternative and find out that there aren't any. Oh well, you figure, you'll just have to do without them.

By the time you're seriously late for your next dose you notice that you're not feeling so great. You're sweating. You feel like ants are crawling all over your skin. You've got diarrhea. So you call your doctor back. He explains that you've become addicted to the pills and that you're going through withdrawal. He also doesn't have anything to help you get through it because tranquilizers haven't been invented. You go *cold turkey*, and, if you survive, and some didn't, you vow never to touch those things again.

All we had done was replace the natural drive to eat with an abnormal drive to use amphetamines.

The backlash against the appetite suppressants was enormous! The public, the medical community, and the public health agencies had all been burned. No one was in a very understanding mood. *Not only were the amphetamines blamed for what happened, but the very idea of using appetite suppressants was condemned.* Attitudes toward weight loss changed again. Once again, people felt that if you wanted to lose weight, you just had to eat less. All you needed was a little will power and a change in attitude to take it off forever. Will power was, once again, the only game in town.

## *The Diet Pills of the Seventies*

Several new, *non-addictive appetite suppressants* were approved in the seventies. For awhile, hope was renewed in the idea of limiting *demand* for food as a means of weight loss, but these medications were doomed by several factors for which they were not to blame.

- The first of these factors was the attitude of the public, the medical community, and the regulators that the medications might be unsafe. The memory of their bad experience with the amphetamines in the thirties was still fresh in everybody's mind in the seventies.

- The second factor was the attitude that appetite suppressants were a crutch, taking the place of will power or self control. Remember that it was not only the amphetamines that were condemned but the entire category of demand limiters as well.

- The third factor was the way in which the regulatory agencies allowed these new medications to be marketed. Understandably concerned about releasing yet another plague upon the land and worried by chemical similarities between the new medications and the amphetamines, the agencies required exhaustive testing prior to approval. Even after the testing showed the medications to be safe and non-addictive, the FDA still imposed two crippling conditions on the information that was supplied with these medications.

- The first condition was that a warning about all of the side effects of amphetamines had to be included, even though research did not find the same problems with the new medications. The medical community was less than enthusiastic about this, and the diet pills were never widely prescribed.

- The final nail in the coffin was the length of time for use specified by the FDA. Their use was approved for only *a few weeks*, giving wary doctors another reason to avoid them and guaranteeing their failure when they were prescribed.

Two of the medications approved under these conditions were phentermine resin, known as Ionamin®, and fenfluramine, known as Pondimin®. With the exception of Redux®, all of the other available appetite suppressants were approved in the same general time frame.

*It has taken **sixty years** after the amphetamine disaster and **twenty years** after the discovery of safe appetite suppressants for us to accept that these new medications are, in fact, safe to use in the treatment of overweight, when used properly. These new medications are the first steps on the road to freedom from overweight.*

Meanwhile, we've been trying to lose weight by going hungry without any success. There's an old saying that nature abhors a vacuum. The vacuum in question was the desire to lose weight without the means to do it. Into the breach stepped the weight loss *industry*.

## CHAPTER 5

# The Weight Loss Industry

With the bad experience of the first demand limiters, the amphetamines, the only avenue of weight loss left to the American public was the diet approach. Diets had been tried since the early years of the twentieth century with the usual rate of success, that is, none. However, the desire for weight loss wasn't changed by the amphetamine experience, only the options available for achieving it.

Literally tens of thousands of diet programs have been offered in the last fifty years. Some of these are honest attempts to search for an effective diet that would work using only will power. Some of them are a little one-sided, suggesting that a leaning in one direction or another, such as protein or carbohydrates might be best. The vast majority of them are downright nuts!

In order to understand just how nuts some diets are, we need to look at some reference point, that is, some basic rules of human nutrition established by the scientific community without the bias of a commercial, religious, astrological, ecological, geological, or psychological agenda. Just what does it take to keep one of us alive and healthy, anyway?

## Basic Human Nutrition

Remember the chapter where we talked about the energy required for all living things? Well, that energy is measured in calories. A calorie is a measure of *energy*, in the form of heat, required to raise the temperature of one gram of pure water one degree centigrade. Note that there are no good calories or bad calories, just calories. We get these calories by digesting food.

Digestion takes complex food molecules like carbohydrates, fats, and proteins and releases energy by breaking them down to their component parts. We can capture the energy released when this is done and pick through the pieces and grab the stuff we need to build our bodies. Pretty neat trick. Oh yes, there are a few more things like vitamins, minerals, trace elements, oxygen, and water necessary for all this to happen, but that's about it. It's really pretty simple unless you want to get into all the gory details and, take it from me, you don't.

## Calorie Requirements

So how many calories do we need? We use up about twenty calories per pound of lean body mass a day. Lean body mass is the weight of everything *but* body fat. So, a man who has 150 pounds of lean body mass uses up about 3,000 calories per day. A woman who has 100 pounds of lean body mass uses up about 2,000 calories per day.

> *In order to lose one pound, a man or woman must burn up 3,500 calories more than he or she consumes.*

**YOU NOW KNOW EVERYTHING YOU HAVE TO KNOW ABOUT LOSING AND GAINING WEIGHT!**

The rules are pretty much the same for everyone as long as they're healthy. Now let's look at how we need to get these calories.

## Carbohydrates, Protein, and Fat

Carbohydrates are easily converted into sugar which is the fuel our cells burn, so we need lots of them for immediate daily consumption. Each gram of carbohydrate contains *four* calories.

Proteins are the building blocks of the structures of our bodies. We need them to replace worn out cells and to repair damage done as we bump into the walls of life. Each gram of protein also contains *four* calories.

We cannot live without some fat in our diet. We need fat because without it we can't absorb the vitamins we need, such as vitamins A, D, E, and K. Fat is also used as building blocks and for energy storage. Each gram of fat contains *nine* calories.

On top of this we need those vitamins, minerals and trace elements I mentioned. Again, that's it.

**The Confusion About Fat**

There is a major point of confusion about fat that needs to be cleared up before we go on. The reason for this confusion is that fat plays a central role in two different issues.

The first issue we'll look at is hardening of the arteries. This process, known as arteriosclerosis, is caused by the accumulation of cholesterol in the lining of the arteries. This results in heart attacks, blockage of the arteries to the legs, and other nasty problems.

Because of the way our bodies make cholesterol, it is important, especially for people with elevated cholesterol, to reduce the amount of fat in their diet. The average American diet gets about 37% of its calories from fat.[20] That's not 37% by weight, or 37% by volume, or 37% by any other measure but calories. The ideal percentage of fat *calories* in the diet is thought by nutritional experts to be less than 30%.[21]

On the other hand, only about 20% of the cholesterol in our bloodstreams comes from cholesterol we eat. We make the other 80% from saturated fats. Saturated fat is one of the forms of fats called triglycerides that we eat. The amount of cholesterol we make from these saturated triglycerides is genetically determined. Those with a family history of high cholesterol need to be especially careful to limit saturated fat. As I tell my patients, if you want good cholesterol numbers, the best thing you can do is choose your parents wisely.

The issue of hardening of the arteries is an important one to our health, but it's not primarily a weight loss issue. A cholesterol problem is diagnosed by a blood test; a weight problem is diagnosed by a mirror and a scale.

The second issue is a weight issue. Fat is *concentrated calories*. Since fat contains, gram for gram, more than twice the calories found in carbohydrates or protein, a little bit of fat contains a lot of calories. Because of this, when we reduce the amount of fat in our diets, we get to eat a lot more food *by weight*, without increasing the amount of calories we're eating. Low-fat diets don't cause weight loss. Low-***calorie*** diets do.

The last bit of complication is caused by the fact that *both* high cholesterol and overweight cause the same risks for some illnesses. Being overweight increases the risk for heart disease *whether or not the individual has high cholesterol*. As a matter of fact, overweight is a risk factor for more problems than high cholesterol.

One of the reasons we eat so much fat probably centers around the issue of satiety. Satiety is the sense of satisfaction we need from our food before we stop eating. Because it takes longer for fat to leave the stomach than carbohydrates or proteins, it's better at making us feel full.[22] In other words, fat treats hunger more effectively than either carbohydrate or protein. It better satisfies the hypothalamus. We can eat rice cakes until our jaws fall off, but we stay hungry and get no *yum* until our hypothalamus signals our brain that *it* is satisfied.

## YOU NOW KNOW EVERYTHING YOU HAVE TO KNOW ABOUT NUTRITION!

Except for the issues surrounding fat, this may seem too simple to a lot of people. The reason for this is that the diet industry can't allow it to remain that simple. We've had decades of *experts* telling us how their approach is best, and, because the facts are too simple, they have to make up new ones to keep the pot boiling. How can you be an *expert* unless you've discovered some new truth you can pass down from on high? If you can't give 'em the *right* answer, you've got to at least dazzle 'em with the footwork. Let's look at the local book store first, then we can look at those TV ads.

There are seventy-two running feet of diet books in the book store nearest to my house. That's seventy-two feet! These books can be broken down into several categories for ease of description.

### *"Just Say No" Diets*

These are based on the idea that dieting is just a mind over matter exercise called will power. These books are full of jewels of wisdom, such as the fact that overweight people eat more fattening foods than thin people . . . what a concept. One author tells us that diets don't work and then tells us how to change our attitude so that we can take in less calories. Last time I looked, that was called a diet. Presumably, if you could just think and feel the right way, you wouldn't *need* to be overweight any more. Sort of a *snap out of it* approach to the problem.

"Hey, Joe, what's the matter? You look glum."

"Oh, hi, Fred. It's 'cause I'm overweight and I can't seem to do anything about it."

"Have you tried eating less?"

"Yeah, but I always end up eating until I'm not hungry, and it seems to result in this weight."

"Hmmm, I see. Hey, I've got an idea. Why don't you eat until you *shouldn't* be hungry, and then convince yourself that you're satisfied. I'll bet you'll lose weight then."

"Wow! Great idea, but what do I do with the hunger that's left over?"

"Uh, go for a walk?"

"Walking makes me hungry."

"How about jogging?"

"Jogging makes me hungry."

"Lose yourself in a good book."

"I get hungry when I read."

"Gee, Joe, you really do have a problem with hunger. I bet if you did something about that, you'd lose some weight."

It's good to have friends who can help you with life's little problems.

### Magic-Food Diets

It seems that specific foods, such as grapefruit, cabbage, kumquats, or beebleberries have some mystical quality that modifies some physical reality. Grapefruit contain little gremlins which crawl into your stomach and prevent you from being hungry. Beebleberries cause the food you eat to fall into another dimension while soothing your hunger with accordion music. Cabbage soup not only smells bad while you cook it, but the resultant gas fills you up and distracts you with thoughts of various musical and not-so-musical notes.

### Special Food Category Diets

These, like the Pritikin diet and the Atkins diet, are based on the idea that if you eat the right category of foods, either the carbohydrates, fats, or proteins, some sort of mystical process will occur whereby your weight loss goals will be reached, your life span will be increased, and you will live happily ever after. Perhaps, if you could get your hypothalamus to read, these might work.

*High-Carbohydrate Diets:* The authors of these diets point out the benefits of carbohydrates over fat or protein. They all reluctantly allow you to eat the *bad* foods but warn you against them. These *experts* tell you that you should eat at least 60% carbohydrates and keep the fat and protein down to 20% each. Sound familiar? The only problem with these diets is that pesky little hunger thing, but supposedly, if you eat the right mixture, you won't be hungry. I think pasta is supposed to coat your hypothalamus and keep it happy.

*High-Protein Diets:* These usually recommend up to 40% protein. The little problems of gout, kidney stress, and the fat almost always associated with protein don't seem to matter to these authors. Other problems associated with high-protein diets include the binding of essential minerals, such as calcium, by excess protein in the bloodstream. This has been identified as one risk for osteoporosis.[23]

*High-Fat Diets*: Yes, folks, there are still a few die-hards out there who haven't figured out that fat is best in moderation. Atkins, in particular, likes to demonstrate his fearlessness on *Oprah* by eating bacon and eggs and all sorts of other greasy goodies. This is supposed to be a high-protein diet, but it sure looked high-fat to me. I won't insult your intelligence by explaining the reasons why this is a bad idea. I suppose the fat makes your hypothalamus slippery so the hunger messages won't stick.

### *Scientific-Discovery Diets*

I specially like the one written by the *expert* who has figured out that insulin is the hormone from hell which causes everything from IRS audits to the heartbreak of psoriasis. This diet reduces the levels of insulin in your body and allows you to be thin. The total lack of a scientific basis for this hypothesis seems to be a minor annoyance.

Another *scientific discovery* is fiber. Supposedly, if you eat enough of the stuff, you will not only lose weight, but you will have lower cholesterol, healthier bowels, and become an accomplished pianist. This falls into the category of "if a little bit is good, a lot is better." Imagine how healthy we'll all be when we eat only hay.

### The Gimmick Diet

Deal-a-meal is my favorite. I'll see your two kumquats and raise you a radish. The rotation diet is another example. If it's Tuesday, it must be chicken breasts. The five-day diet only keeps you hungry for five days at a time.

### The Street-Sign Diet

"Lose 30 pounds in 30 days for $30!" Hmm, let's see, you need to eat 3,500 calories less than you burn to lose one pound. That means that you'll have to burn up 4,500 calories a day on a 1,000 calorie diet to lose one pound a day. I'll bet this diet involves the use of either a machete or a blowtorch! Makes sense to me.

Now let's look at the TV ads.

"Give us a week and we'll take off the weight!" Right! And if we manage to go hungry for the whole week, give us another one and we'll put it right back on.

Weight Watchers™ offers an excellent, well-designed diet, much like the one I use in my program. Now about that little hunger thing . . .

Another program offers to take it all off for a dollar a pound. They'll also sell you all of the food you eat, and, if you eat only their food, you'll be guaranteed to lose weight. All you have to do is pay them for your food forever and stay hungry all the time and your problem is solved.

### *The Common Denominator*

These represent a small fraction of the kinds of diets out there. But I'll let you look for yourself after you finish this book. Remember, it's impolite to laugh unless you've got a copy of this book in your hands.

All of these diets have two things in common. These *experts* are not stupid. They all reduce the level of caloric intake, and they all produce weight loss *as long as they are followed.* That's the key.

> **It's not the special characteristic of the diet that causes weight loss.**
> **It's the reduction in calories.**

They have a second common characteristic:

> **All diets ask people to do something they can't do in the long haul ... go hungry.**

None of them are effective in dealing with the hunger that inevitably happens when you reduce the number of calories you eat. The result of this minor detail is that the success rates of these diets is somewhere between dismal and zero.

### Of all people who lose weight on diets alone, 95% put the weight back on within three years.

The next question is how many people don't lose weight at all? The true success rate of diets has been estimated to be as low as 0.5%!

*That means that one out of every two hundred people who go on a diet will lose a significant amount of weight and keep it off.* These are seriously lousy odds.

The weight loss industry has succeeded *because* it hasn't come up with the answer to overweight. As long as there are people who want to lose weight, there will always be someone who hasn't heard that a particular diet doesn't work. Those *thirty-five BILLION dollars* will continue to be spent every year in search of the holy grail of the magic diet, the one that can take it off and keep it off.

We have not failed the weight loss industry. The weight loss industry has failed us. It has led us to believe that the answers it was *selling* were handed down from on high and proven by experience. At no time did any of these *experts* dare to subject any of their theories to the cold light of scientific evaluation, nor is there any federal regulatory agency, like the FDA, that requires them to do so. As a result, they can claim almost anything. What would happen if they gave you the facts? Imagine a sign placed over the diet books in your book store.

***Up to 5% success rate by some studies
(Up to 0.5% in others)***

***All diets in this section unproven and none
objectively evaluated.***

***The author makes no representations
as to the effectiveness of any of these diets.***

The weight loss industry has shackled us with the blame for *its* failures. After all, it must be our fault. We must be doing something to cause all of these failures because, even when we're shown THE ANSWER by some *expert* in the field of writing diet books, we can't seem to control ourselves.

We need to free ourselves from this trap and allow the blame for failure to rest where it belongs, squarely on the shoulders of those who have failed to understand the nature of the problem and who have profited from our attempts to follow their answers.

The field of psychology has also become an unwilling accomplice in the blame game.

## CHAPTER 6

# The Misuse of Psychology In Weight Loss

With the growth of psychology in the fifties and sixties came new ways of looking at the problem of being overweight. Various factions of the growing field had their own view as to its causes.

The Freudians and Jungians decided that the desire for food was just a metaphor for the sex drive. The desire for food was also associated with the "oral fixation" presumably caused by weaning too early.

The behaviorists concluded that the problem was eating behaviors learned in childhood. They suggested that by changing behaviors related to eating, such as driving to work a different way so that you don't pass the doughnut shop or only eating at the dining room table, you would find it easy to lose weight. It didn't turn out to be that easy.

The "new age" psychologists suggested that we should get in touch with our *inner selves* so that we could understand our motivations and stop eating. They recommended activities, such as meditation, to overcome the appetite. Meditation may have helped to relieve some stress in a fast-paced world, but it was not the answer to overweight.

One particularly offensive idea propounded by some psychologists is that some women become overweight in order to become unattractive to men. This is a blatant case of explaining observations in terms of the prejudices of the observer.

The different psychological theories surrounding the overweight problem remind me of the often-told story of the blind men and the elephant.

> It seems that there were several blind men standing around an elephant trying to figure out what it was. One man, standing near the trunk, said it was a snake with a strange mouth; another man, at the tail, said it was a vine; another, at a leg, said it was a tree trunk; and another, at an ear, said it was a huge leaf. When they compared notes, they concluded that they had found a large tree, with huge leaves, with vines growing on it, containing a snake.

Unhampered by the facts, they were free to make the data fit their preconceived ideas.

Of course, the weight loss *experts* in the industry saw all of this psychological stuff as manna from heaven because it kept the public from realizing the truth about their lack of success. Failure of the *experts'* programs could be blamed on factors that were impossible to disprove. There were now all sorts of psychological reasons why people didn't succeed, such as "negative self talk" and "fear of being thin."

The industry viewed overweight as a result of stress, guilt, loneliness, fear, or anxiety, and, presumably, if we could just get rid of those feelings, we wouldn't need to eat. They were right that eating was caused by a feeling, but they were blaming it on the wrong one. The feeling that causes us to eat is *hunger*, and the important point is this:

## Hunger is not under conscious control.

Hunger is controlled by the hypothalamus, which is also a major control center for the expression of emotion in terms of behavior. In times of stress, one of the things that the hypothalamus does is to increase the appetite in overweight people and to decrease the appetite in thin people. Which one happens is determined by circumstances at least partly genetic in nature.

Emotionally-induced hunger is what is called a threshold event. Once the behavior is triggered, it will play itself out to its natural conclusion. The emotionally upset person eating an ice cream is like a cat in the middle of a cat fight. If you try to intervene during the fight, you'll get yourself bitten. Only after the adrenaline wears off, in the case of the cat, or after the serotonin is released, in the case of the human, can reason take hold. The point is:

### If you block the hunger signal with medication, the hypothalamus no longer gets to control our behavior.

The bottom line is that the hypothalamus is controlling *hunger,* a hunger not under the conscious control of the human being. Psychological factors don't cause overweight. They cause *hunger* which *causes* overweight. The result of all this is:

### It is impossible to assess the importance of psychological factors in causing overweight until hunger is effectively turned off in the brain.

> I like the story about a guy who goes to a psychiatrist because he thinks he might have a multiple personality disorder. The psychiatrist listens to him for about five minutes and states that he is certain that the patient doesn't have more than one personality. When the patient asks the psychiatrist how he can be so sure so quickly, the psychiatrist answers that he's certain that if the patient had more than one personality he wouldn't use the one he was using.

If we had a choice, we wouldn't be overweight. It's something that happens to us like high blood pressure or appendicitis. People don't wake up one morning, look in the mirror, and decide that they're going to put on some weight. If we had a choice, we'd all be our ideal, healthy weight forever.

The point is:

**Overweight is not a psychological issue.
It's a biological issue.**

CHAPTER 7

# The Misunderstanding of Exercise in Weight Loss

How many times have you heard, or said, "No matter how much I exercise, I just can't seem to lose any weight?" I've been told the same thing by literally hundreds of patients, almost all of them women. I used to think that these women were exaggerating until I observed the phenomenon for myself.

About ten years ago, my wife and I exercised regularly at a local aerobics studio. I was able to lose about twenty pounds by combining a sensible diet with my exercise. My wife was able to lose about eight pounds by doing the same. We met a lady in our class who obviously needed to take off some weight. She attended at least as regularly as we did and worked hard at her exercise but didn't seem to be losing any weight. There was an important reason why.

A fascinating study[24] was done using two groups of young, healthy, female, university students. Both of these groups were sedentary, that is non-exercising, by nature. One group began to run fifteen miles per week on a regular basis, and the other group actually began training for a marathon run. No effort was made by either group to change their dietary habits. In both groups there was *absolutely no weight loss*!

There are two reasons for this. The first is that women have less muscle mass than men relative to their total body weight. Since it's the muscle that burns calories, women burn fewer calories than men during exercise.

The second reason is hormonal. One of the female hormones, progesterone, promotes the storage of fat and the use of carbohydrates during exercise. Testosterone, the male hormone, promotes the burning of fat with exercise. Because of this, women's bodies will use up all the available carbohydrates before they begin to burn fat. Unless there's a shortage of the preferred fuel, carbohydrates, fat will not be mobilized and consumed. Women need to be carbohydrate depleted *before* they exercise in order to burn fat.

Mother Nature has made men sprinters, ready to use up all our available resources in the short run. Women were designed to be around for the long haul to grow and birth babies. They need to be able to save up energy for the really important work, like keeping the species going. Because of this:

**While exercise alone causes weight loss in men, exercise alone is ineffective for weight loss in women.[25] In order to lose weight with exercise, women must combine exercise with reduction of caloric intake.**

That doesn't mean that women shouldn't exercise. Exercise is important for several reasons:

- The commitment to exercise is a critical part of the commitment to a healthier life style. It's a mistake to think that all you have to do to keep the weight off is take diet pills. Remember, the results show that the pills work in combination with modification of diet, behavior, *and exercise.*

- Exercise creates a sense of wellness and control over one's body. The importance of this benefit cannot be emphasized enough. Muscle strength, balance, and loss of fear of physical risk is essential in promoting a sense of wellness. Your body really follows the principle of *use it or lose it.* If it doesn't need to preserve something because it isn't being used, that something will usually go away.

- Exercise tones muscles, and toning muscles has tremendous cosmetic value. Muscles used to being stretched over fat won't tighten up by themselves. The current ideal of the beautiful woman or man is defined by the muscle shape and not by the shape of the fat layer over that muscle.

- Exercise reduces LDL cholesterol, which causes hardening of the arteries, and increases HDL cholesterol, which protects against hardening of the arteries.[26]

- Aerobic exercise has important cardiopulmonary benefits as proven by Kenneth Cooper, MD, in his excellent studies in Dallas. These studies show that exercise increases the capacity of the heart and lungs to use oxygen. This creates two extremely important benefits to the exerciser.

  The first is that your body becomes a more efficient *furnace*. The number of calories you burn in your furnace is directly related to how much oxygen you can get to the fire. Aerobic exercise brings more oxygen into the system which burns more calories.[27]

  The second benefit is that exercise increases circulation to the heart and lungs. Heart attacks are caused by a lack of blood supply to the heart muscle, and exercise increases the blood supply available.[28]

Both men *and* women get all of these benefits from exercise, but only men effectively lose weight from exercise alone.

By the way, the story of our fellow exerciser has a happy ending. She obviously figured out how to realize her goals in more ways than one. That lady is Susan Powter, author of *Stop the Insanity*.

One of the definitions of insanity is doing the same thing time after time and expecting a different outcome each time you do it. Susan realized that diets *alone* don't work and identified exercise as the other necessary component. To an extent, she's right. But I feel that the level of exercise necessary to maintain weight loss, along with the hunger endured without appetite suppressants, will still fail in the long run for the vast majority of us. For example, when my wife and I stopped doing aerobics, we regained the weight. Like the majority of people, we just couldn't maintain the level of exercise necessary to maintain the weight loss. The resulting weight gain is inevitable without some kind of permanent help.

One of the basic elements of my weight loss program is to negotiate a program of exercise with each person. I use the term negotiate, because it's useless to try to dictate exercise to someone who just doesn't want to do it. The minimum exercise plan I recommend is walking twenty minutes, three times a week. Exercise is important for all the reasons I mentioned, but I don't depend on it to help my patients lose weight.

## Reduction in calories is what gets results. Weight lost by exercising is a bonus.

So what does this mean in practical terms? If you are female, it means that you can't depend on exercise alone to lose weight. But, if you exercise while reducing calories with the help of an appetite suppressant, the benefits in terms of added weight loss and improvement in health are clear. If you are male, exercise alone will help, but it's not the only answer.

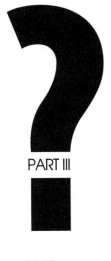

# PART III

# What To Do About It

# CHAPTER 8
# How Does All This Apply To You?

Let's use Lynn as our example of a weight loss patient. This forty-year-old lady has been trying to lose forty pounds for about twenty years. She's tried every resource available and has lost a grand total of about 120 pounds on different diets only to regain it all once she stopped dieting. She hasn't quite given up, but she has been bitten so often by the weight loss monster that she feels like a teething ring, and she's shown up to see if we have anything to offer her she hasn't tried. It's my job to convince her that everything she thinks she knows about being overweight is wrong and to get her on the right track.

Lynn is convinced that her weight is at an "unnatural" level and that underneath it there is the 120-pound, twenty-year-old girl she used to be, just waiting to be liberated. She admits that most of the women in her family go through the same weight changes with the passage of time and childbearing, but she doesn't understand why her efforts to change have failed.

I begin by explaining to Lynn that her present weight is her *natural* weight. She isn't very happy about this at first, because it sounds like I'm telling her that she doesn't have a problem. But I go on to explain that this is not her healthy weight nor is it the weight at which she feels comfortable and has the best self esteem. Still, it is her *natural* weight.

When I explain that this is her natural weight because she's been doing what comes naturally, that is, satisfying her hunger, she begins to understand.

When I explain that hunger is not something humans can control or ignore, she begins to understand why will power has never worked for her. It hasn't worked *because* she is a normal human being.

The final key to Lynn's understanding is helping her to see that she is fulfilling her genetic destiny just like all of the other women in her family. Not all people have obvious family traits of overweight, but genetics plays a part whether or not that part is obvious.

"But the reason I'm overweight is that I eat when I'm *not* hungry."

People experience hunger in different ways. There is the feeling of "emptiness" as the stomach growls which we all call hunger. But there is also the quiet voice of nature reminding us that we need to store up for the winter. This is the voice we hear when we're "bored," or not actively involved in something interesting or important enough to drown it out. It's still hunger, but it's a different kind of signal. Hunger is the urge to eat. There are different causes and types, but they're all hunger.

"But I eat when I'm angry, or frustrated, or whenever I feel some strong emotion. How can I ever hope to keep the weight off unless I become a hermit?"

The hunger signals your brain gets are increased by emotions, but they're still hunger signals. We don't eat because we're upset, we eat because being upset makes us *hungry*. This is one of the most powerful types of hunger that there is.

"But I eat all the wrong foods. I love sweets and fatty food, and I just can't get myself to eat fruits and vegetables all the time."

All you're saying is that it takes a certain number of calories to turn off your hunger once it gets turned on. Of course your personal tastes will dictate that you get these calories in the most pleasant way you can. The primary goal of the hunger urge is satisfaction, and as long as you're driven by the urge you won't be able to make wise choices. You'll be too busy trying to satisfy your hunger.

Lynn, your problem with overweight just isn't your fault. There's absolutely nothing *wrong* with you. The problem is that when you behave in a natural way you end up overweight. All of the reasons for *your* failures are excuses your previous programs have given you for *their* failure. You are a natural woman doing exactly what you are supposed to do and being blamed for doing it.

"No one has ever talked to me about my weight like this before. I've always been blamed for my failure to be thin. You mean it's not my fault?"

Your weight is no more your *fault* than the color of your eyes, the shape of your hands, or your height are. All you are doing is the best you can with the hand that Mother Nature dealt you.

"So how do I get around Mother Nature's plan for me?"

We've got to outwit Mother Nature by making her think that you are following her instructions. We do this by using appetite suppressants.

"I know all about those weight loss pills. They're all "speed," and those speed pills will kill you and make you an addict. My grandfather told me all about his sister who got hooked on them back in the thirties. She swore she'd rather die then go through that again."

Those were the amphetamines, and your family's experience was typical. The newer appetite suppressants don't cause addiction and are safe to take under a doctor's supervision.

"If they're so safe then why are they approved for only a few weeks use?"

These medications were approved back in the seventies when the regulatory agencies were still frightened by the experience people like your family had with the amphetamines in the thirties. In May of 1996, these same agencies approved a new appetite suppressant called Redux®, for indefinite use. Redux® is no more effective or any safer than the appetite suppressants we've had since the seventies.

"I guess these regulators have finally realized that a person has a right to look as good as she or he wants to."

It's not the cosmetic value of thinness that dictated the new attitude of the regulators. It was the realization that overweight is one of the biggest health risk factors in this country today. They realized that a certain amount of risk is acceptable to treat some levels of overweight just as some risk is acceptable to treat all of the *consequences* of overweight like heart disease, diabetes, and some forms of cancer.

"How long do I have to take these pills before my stomach shrinks and I can stop them?"

Expecting your stomach to shrink from eating less food is like expecting your need for oxygen to go away if you breathe less deeply. It doesn't work that way. The studies have shown that as soon as you stop the pills the weight comes right back.

"You mean to tell me that you want me to take these things for the rest of my life? I'm already taking pills for high blood pressure, and diabetes runs in my family.

I'm going to look like a drug store. I'm not crazy about the idea of taking pills in the first place."

That's the point. Overweight is an underlying risk factor for those very diseases. Wouldn't you rather treat the underlying risk factor than the diseases that result from it? It's even possible that you won't need to take your blood pressure medication after you've lost weight.

Do you recognize anyone you know in Lynn? Yourself perhaps? Lynn's concerns are a product of the information given to her by the diet industry and are perfectly understandable in that context. Her concerns about the appetite suppressants are perfectly reasonable, given her own family's experiences with the amphetamines. There's nothing wrong with Lynn's thinking. She's just using old and inaccurate information.

Lynn decides to try the appetite suppressants. She remains somewhat skeptical, but she's tried everything else and failed, and she feels she's got nothing to lose. Her attitude is "show me." She starts her medication to suppress her appetite, and she turns out to be one of the good responders with few, if any, side effects and good therapeutic results.

It's now one month later and she's lost eight pounds. Lynn has been here before. She's had the experience of initial success. As a matter of fact, she's even done better on one of those liquid protein diets. But there's a difference. Lynn no longer craves food! She can stare the cakes and cookies and cheeseburgers right in the face and feel nothing. She can go to a party and, when her friend loads her up a plate of her favorite many-layered bean dip and chips, she can take a bite, enjoy the flavor, and put the rest down. It is completely unnecessary for her to "fill up" to enjoy the food.

Lynn now understands why this program works so well. She is free of the hunger she has always had to deal with on her previous diets. She is free of the guilt for being overweight in the first place. She is also free of the fear that her weight will return as soon as she lets down her guard. Most importantly Lynn is free to see herself as a good, strong person whose weight is just a management problem, not a reflection of her worth.

Lynn's success on her program isn't just a matter of her taking appetite suppressants. All of the studies show the same results; these medications work when they are combined with a proper program of diet and exercise. The next question is, what constitutes a proper program?

# CHAPTER 9

# An Ethical Weight Loss Program

Let's assume that you've decided to use the information in this book to find a weight loss program. The first challenge you have is to find one which is ethical. Ethical means that the program is designed primarily with your interests and safety in mind, and not the convenience, comfort, or profit of the people running the program.

The four elements of an ethical weight loss program are:

- Evaluation and examination
- Program design
- Informed consent
- Follow-up

While there are no strict rules as to how each of these components should be implemented, each one is essential to ensure that your program is safe and effective.

## *Evaluation and Examination*

This is the process of finding out whether you can safely participate in a weight loss program. The first step is to determine whether the benefits of weight loss *from a medical point of view* outweigh the risks associated with a program *enough to justify* your exposure to those risks. Those benefits depend on several things. These are:

- How much weight do you need to lose?
- How old are you?
- What is your past medical history?
- What is your past weight loss history?
- Are there any special considerations that need to be taken into account in the design of your program, such as medications you are taking, allergies, or other special needs?
- What is your present medical condition?

## *Program Design*

There are as many programs as there are people. Each individual's program should be designed with the needs of that particular individual in mind. The elements of program design are:

- Choice of appetite suppressant(s)
- Diet
- Nutritional supplements
- Exercise

## *Informed Consent*

How can you be asked to take the risks of a weight loss program when you don't know what those risks are? How can you evaluate the benefits without knowing what they are?

Informed consent involves your doctor's honest disclosure of:

- The chances of success on the selected program when known and the disclosure that they are not known when this is the case.
- The general risks of any weight loss program.
- The risks associated with the use of the appetite suppressants selected.
- The risks associated with other elements of the selected program such as exercise or nutritional supplements.

## *Follow-Up*

Follow-up is one of the most important safety features in any program. Your doctor must evaluate your progress as long as you are in your program to ensure your safety and the program's effectiveness.

At each follow-up visit, your doctor should assess your:

- Level of hunger
- Amount of weight change
- Health status
- Medication side effects
- Compliance taking the medications

## *Selecting an Ethical Weight Loss Program*

When you're looking for a weight loss program, make sure all four elements of an ethical program are present. Don't be afraid to ask the doctor or his or her staff about every issue. They should be as prepared to address your concerns as they are to accept your payment. If all you get are blank stares, or evasive answers, run, do not walk, to the nearest exit and continue your search.

In the next chapters, we'll look at each of the four elements in more detail.

CHAPTER 10

# Evaluation and Examination

The goal of your evaluation and examination is to answer a number of important questions about you, your health, and your weight loss goals. The answer to these questions will help you and your doctor decide whether the benefits of weight loss from a medical point of view outweigh the risks associated with a program enough to justify your exposure to those risks.

Let's begin by answering one of several important questions.

***How much weight do you need to lose?***

This is not just a matter of putting you on a scale, measuring your height, and plugging the results into a table made up by some insurance company. This is a serious medical question that needs an objective answer. One of the ways to get that answer is to measure your lean body mass. Your lean body mass is the weight of everything *but* the fat in your body.

To determine your lean body mass, I use an impedance meter. This device measures the electrical impedance of your body. It's about the size of a calculator and has two electrodes that are placed on one foot and two that are placed on the wrist on the same side of your body.

The software that comes with the impedance meter takes this measurement along with your weight, height, age and sex, and produces an accurate assessment of your lean body mass and the amount of fat on your body. As a general guideline, a woman should have a maximum of between 22% and 27% of her weight as fat, and a man should have between 13% and 18%, depending on age.[29] With this information I can calculate how much fat you should have on your body and *objectively* evaluate your weight.

There is no way for me to assess the benefits of a weight loss program and the acceptable risks without this measurement. There is also no other objective way for me to tell a patient that she doesn't need to lose weight without getting my head chewed off. (It has never, so far, happened with a man.) Let me tell you about one such incident.

# Evaluation And Examination

I offer a free weight loss consult to prospective patients. I walked into an examining room one day to do a consultation and I immediately realized that I had a problem. Sitting in the patient's chair was a twenty-two-year-old woman wearing a halter top and shorts which revealed a flat abdomen and thin arms. This young woman was ready to sign up for a weight loss program right then and there, no questions asked.

We talked about the risks of appetite suppressants for a few minutes, and I offered to objectively evaluate her body composition to see whether those risks would be acceptable in her case.

When we got the results of the test back it turned out that she had a body fat of 18%. This was at the *lower* limit of the normal range for her and she was delighted. All she really needed was some reassurance that she was not overweight. If I had tried to give her verbal reassurance it would have meant less than nothing to her. I would have been a male person telling her that she looked good to me. With the data on her body mass I become a doctor evaluating her condition.

## *How old are you?*

The evaluation process must be modified in people under the age of eighteen. One of the most important considerations is whether it is the patient or a parent who wants the weight loss. As the father of four, I am experienced enough to know that a teenager isn't going to do anything he or she doesn't want to do. If it turns out that weight loss is the young person's agenda, I evaluate the maturity of the patient and the dynamics of the family.

A mature young person in a supportive family has a good chance of success on this program. An immature or angry young person embroiled in an unsupportive family situation may use the weight loss program either as one more point of contention or as a means of self-destructive behavior.

I don't have a set lower age limit for inclusion, but I don't think there are many kids under the age of twelve who'd qualify.

The other end of the age spectrum has it's own considerations. Many people over the age of sixty have other health issues to be dealt with in addition to their weight. The evaluation process is often more detailed in older people and sometimes includes consultation with other doctors who might be looking after the patient.

### *What is your medical history?*

The risks of a weight loss program have to be evaluated for each individual patient. Your current and past medical history will provide important information about any special risks to be considered when a program is designed for you. A history of high blood pressure, diabetes, gall bladder disease, or heart disease, to name a few, will change the design of your program. Donna is a case in point.

> Donna first came to my office when she was referred by her employer for whom she works as a nanny.

Donna weighed three hundred and sixty-five pounds. She is five foot three inches tall and is forty-two years old.

Donna had been taking a medication to make her heart beat more strongly as well as a diuretic to deal with the heart failure caused by her extreme overweight. For reasons only known to her, Donna decided that she didn't need those pills any more and stopped taking them. When I saw her she was unable to walk ten feet without getting short of breath.

After I put her back on her medications, Donna was again able to carry on with her daily activities, but I explained to her that unless she did something about her weight, she could expect her heart to last her only a few more years. Donna decided to do just that, and she is now south of three hundred pounds for the first time in fifteen years.

Donna's history of congestive heart failure, coupled with the enlargement of her heart which occurred as a consequence of it, played a major part in the design of her program. Without knowing how severe her problem was, I could have made her worse instead of better. The dosage of her medication, the design of her exercise, the speed of her weight loss, and the kind of follow up all had to be modified to take Donna's risks into account.

### ***What is your past weight loss history?***

What has worked best for you in the past? What kinds of problems did you have that we can prevent in this program? What are your expectations and beliefs about weight loss? Are you still blaming yourself for the failure of those past programs?

Although this program will be different from your past experiences, old beliefs can get in the way of your success if you don't deal with them directly. Let's look at Joyce as an example.

> Joyce came to my office for the first recheck on her new program. Joyce is an executive with a medical company who travels extensively and who is used to being in control of her environment. Her ongoing weight problem has been a source of frustration for her especially because of her type A personality. It's one of the few areas of her life that she hasn't been able to manage.
>
> Joyce had lost seven pounds in her first week, and I expressed concern as to whether she was eating all of the food in her diet. She assured me that she was, and that, apart from some sleeplessness and some hot flashes, she felt fine. I explained to Joyce that the sleeplessness was probably a side effect of her medication, and that if it didn't go away we might have to change the timing or the dosage of her appetite suppressant. When she was asked about the hot flashes Joyce admitted to stopping her hormone pills. She said that she had gained weight when she started them, and she was bound and determined that *nothing* was going to interfere with this weight loss program. "I've failed at so many diets that I'm not going to take any chances with this one."
>
> My first response to Joyce was that she had *not* failed on her previous diets, and that, in spite of the fact

that they had asked her to do something that she as a human being could not do, that is go hungry, she had managed to lose weight on all of them, only to put it all back on. The failure was on the part of the diets which had failed to recognize her nature as a human being.

My second response was to explain to Joyce that taking her hormones is a quality of life issue, just like her weight. Because the appetite suppressants work on the brain, the increased hunger caused by her hormones should not conflict with her weight loss program. It's not acceptable for her to have to give up the cardiac, bone, and sexual benefits of hormones in order to lose weight. The aim of my program is wellness, not just weight loss.

Joyce was relieved and agreed to take her hormones. She didn't lose much weight her next visit since she put back on the water weight she lost by stopping her hormones, but I explained to her that she had still lost weight even if the scale didn't show it.

Joyce's weight loss history was one of the primary factors in setting her expectations of the program.

### ***What medications are you taking?***

This program is about suppressing the appetite with medication. These medications need to be prescribed in such a way so that they are safe in combination with your existing medications. Allergies, sensitivities, and any unusual responses to other medications need to be assessed as well.

## *What is your present medical condition?*

The only way to answer this question is to do an examination. This includes an electrocardiogram, urinalysis, blood count, biochemical evaluation which includes a blood sugar, electrolyte evaluation, bone metabolism evaluation, iron level, enzyme measurements to determine the health of your internal organs, and a thorough quantitative and qualitative evaluation of your cholesterol, a thyroid evaluation, and a physical exam. Just in case you think that this is overkill, let me tell you about Sam.

> Sam is a thirty-two-year-old car salesman who came to my program as an established patient. His parents, brothers, wife, and daughter are also my patients. Sam decided that it was time for him and his wife to take off their excess weight since his mother had lost fifty pounds on the program.
>
> Because Sam had been a patient of mine since the age of about seventeen, I wasn't expecting there to be any problem with his physical, but when I reviewed his electrocardiogram it turned out that he had a condition called Wolff Parkinson White Syndrome. This is caused by the development of an abnormal electrical conduction pathway in the heart, and can result in the sudden onset of a fast heart rate and sudden cardiac death. This is not the kind of condition you want someone to have who is going to be placed on appetite suppressants. Needless to say, Sam had the abnormality in his heart fixed before we even considered his weight.
>
> Addie is another case in point. She turned out to have an underactive thyroid gland. That wasn't the cause

of her overweight since comparison with previous tests done by her family doctor showed that this was a new problem which was just beginning to happen. Imagine putting Addie on appetite suppressants and watching as nothing happened. That's what would have happened as her metabolism came to a halt when her thyroid failed. After the problem was taken care of she did well on the program.

Only after the process of evaluation and examination is finished can a program be designed for you that takes into account your individual needs. Having reached this point we can now begin to design that program.

# CHAPTER 11

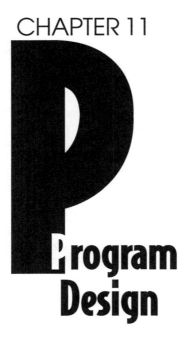

# Program Design

Appetite suppressants work most effectively in conjunction with a program of diet and exercise. I also strongly recommend the use of nutritional supplements in my program. All these elements should be designed specifically for your situation based on your examination and evaluation. The first part of designing your program is the choice of your appetite suppressant.

### Appetite Suppressants

Remember that the program is *not* about appetite **suppressants**, it's about appetite **suppression**, so the key is to find which appetite suppressants work best for you. It doesn't really matter which one turns out to be right for you as long as it works. This means that it might take some trial and error to find the right one. You should also be aware that it might be necessary to change your appetite suppressant after you've been on the program for some time. This happens because the medications can lose their effectiveness after a while. Just because a particular medication gets you on the road doesn't mean it's going to get you all the way to your destination. Both you and your doctor need to keep a close watch on your hunger as you progress and make any necessary adjustments in your program.

Program design has to remain flexible in order to take into account the needs of the individual patient. The first question to be considered is how much weight do you need to lose?

## **_What if I need to lose less than 10% of my body weight?_**

There are many people who want to lose ten or fifteen pounds in order to feel better about themselves. Many people and doctors dismiss these people's concerns as being frivolous, or "just" cosmetic, but to the person in question that ten pounds may be just as important as the fifty pounds others have to lose. Once all is said and done, overweight is a quality of life issue. The most important judge of you is you. The same principles apply to you as apply to the very overweight, that is, will power doesn't work. In my opinion, if you need to lose less than 10% of your body weight, you are not sufficiently overweight to be exposed to the risks of the prescription appetite suppressants. In these cases, I recommend the use of the quick release form of an over-the-counter appetite suppressant called phenylpropanolamine, or PPA for short. PPA is described in more detail in Appendix A.

For some people, PPA will not work effectively and for others, PPA may work too well. Some people may have such effective appetite suppression that they are in danger of malnutrition. That's why it's so important to be in a program monitored by a doctor even when the medication is available over the counter. It is imperative that you lose weight at a safe rate. Also, without a complete program people tend to go back to their old eating habits once the weight starts coming off.

## ***What if I need to lose more than 10% of my body weight?***

Generally, if you need to lose at least 10% of your present body weight, I would recommend the use of a prescription appetite suppressant. For example, if you are a 200 pound man your goal weight must be below 180 pounds. If you are a 150 pound woman then your goal weight must be below 135 pounds. If you are under the age of eighteen, you would need to lose 20% of your present body weight to use a prescription appetite suppressant because of the increased risks of weight loss in young people.

The choice of which prescription appetite suppressants is one of the most difficult ones I have to make. That's not because of the dangers of the medications but because of the lack of long-term research on their effectiveness.

In spite of their association with a rare but serious side effect, Primary Pulmonary Hypertension, (see Appendix A), my first recommendations are usually the use of phentermine (Ionamin®) and fenfluramine (Pondimin®) or dexfenfluramine (Redux®). These are my first choices because they are the only medications in which adequate studies have been done on their long-term effectiveness. I know the other ones work and are reasonably safe, but I have no idea what percent of the people will respond to them or for how long they will work. The reason for this uncertainty is the way the research was done on the appetite suppressants that were introduced in the seventies.

Until the health risks of overweight became known, the whole idea of appetite suppression was not taken seriously by the medical and regulatory communities. It was seen as giving in to the public desire for a cosmetic "quick fix." Because of this, the researchers didn't bother to do studies for more than the required three-month period. All that the research was designed to do was show that the medication in question was superior to a placebo. A typical research paper might be summarized like this:

> "Substance x resulted in a weight loss of an average of 32 pounds over a period of three months in an average of 175 people, whereas the placebo resulted in a weight loss of only 8 pounds in the same period. This is a statistically significant difference and establishes the fact that substance x is an effective appetite suppressant."

Note that there is no information on how long substance x will be effective or whether twenty percent or fifty percent or eighty percent of the people who took it had good results. The average amount of weight loss is a valuable measurement, but it's not enough data to predict the effectiveness of the medication in a long-term program. That's what makes the Weintraub study of phen fen so important. This was the first report on the clinical effectiveness of the appetite suppressants. It was also the first report that addressed effectiveness as if it mattered to the health of the patient.

The four year length of the Weintraub study[30] was also a first for the appetite suppressants, again a reflection of the fact that overweight is a long-term problem that needs to be treated long term.

What the Weintraub study showed was that the combination of phentermine resin, known as Ionamin®, and dl fenfluramine, known as Pondimin® was:

- effective in causing more than 10% weight loss for up to three years in up to 40% of the people in the study when used in combination with a program of diet and exercise and behavior modification.
- well tolerated by 90% of the patients. Only 10% dropped out because of medication side effects.
- safe in this study. All of the observed side effects went away when the medication was stopped and none were dangerous.
- not addictive, with no behavior of any patients suggesting tolerance or abuse.
- effective as long as it was used. People's stomachs don't "shrink." As soon as the medications were stopped, people regained all of their weight.

Contrast these findings with the studies done on each of the two medications separately in the seventies. These showed that they worked better than a placebo.

The studies done on dexfenfluramine, known as Redux® were of the Weintraub type, and I expect that new studies will be done on the other available appetite suppressants to show their clinical effectiveness as well. The individual appetite suppressants are described in Appendix A.

### *Diet*

Diet is a key part of your weight loss program. When all is said and done, the entire program centers around giving you the ability to modify the way you eat for the rest of your life. Unless this part is done right, it's all a waste of your time. Suppressing your appetite allows you to achieve that goal.

Although there are a number of ways to design a diet just for you, I have chosen to use the computer program that comes with the impedance meter that I use to calculate lean body mass. This program gives diet "experts" like me the ability to design your diet without having to consult a nutritionist.

Once the amount of your lean body mass is measured, the program calculates your total daily calorie usage. This will be the sum of:

- Your basal metabolic rate
- The calories you burn digesting food
- The calories you use in your daily activities
- The calories you burn exercising

The program is designed to create a 1,000 calorie per day deficit which will result in a weight loss of two pounds per week (3,500 calories per pound, 7,000 calories per week). In the case of a small woman, it will not create a dietary plan of less than 1,000 calories per day, and, in the case of a large man, it may design a diet which will cause up to a three pound a week loss. It's designed with safety in mind, not weight loss at any cost.

The program then designs a diet which consists of 60% carbohydrate, 20% protein, and 20% fat and breaks it down into an exchange diet similar to the one used by Weight Watchers™. It also calculates the amount of cholesterol, sodium, and fiber in your diet.

The ability of your doctor to modify the program to take into account any special dietary needs you may have is the final safety feature designed into the software. This is one of the areas where the evaluation of special needs such as your age and your medical history can be taken into account. For instance, in the case of patients under the age of eighteen, I increase the amount of protein to 30% with just a few key strokes on the computer.

Your dietary plan will also be used to make sure you are eating enough food. When the medications work well, some people will actually stop eating altogether and will be at risk for malnutrition. This is a potentially serious side effect of demand limitation and can only be prevented by proper dietary design. If I don't know how much you're supposed to lose in a given period of time, I can't tell whether you're eating properly.

There are other ways to accomplish all this without a computer program. But unless medical education has changed, and I know it hasn't changed that much, a computer program like the one I use is the only way most doctors will be able to easily include all of these variables to customize your program.

### *Exercise*

One of the basic elements of your weight loss program should be exercise. I try to negotiate a program of exercise with everyone in my program, but I don't depend on it to help them lose weight. Some of us just don't like to exercise and there's no sense beginning any weight loss program with a lie. I'm going to encourage you to exercise throughout your program, but I'm not going to make it an issue between us. Exercise needs to be individualized according to the individual's age, medical history, and personal preferences.

One of the pieces of information that my software program must have in order to calculate your diet is the daily caloric value of exercise you agree to do. It offers choices from walking to cross country skiing, as well as detailed weight lifting data. Some of my patients only burn off an extra thirty calories a day with exercise, and others use exercise to burn off up to five hundred calories a day. The minimum exercise plan I recommend is walking twenty minutes three times a week.

### *Nutritional Supplements*

Nutritional supplements contain substances which are not made by our own bodies but which are necessary for good health. They include the vitamins, the minerals, and fiber.

Vitamins are necessary for life but are not produced by our own bodies. They are vital for the production of the components of our bodies as well as the for the metabolic functions necessary for life.

Minerals such as copper, zinc, magnesium, and chromium, are necessary for the normal function of many of the enzymes in our bodies. Calcium is vital for bone health as well as normal muscle function, and iron is essential for the formation of hemoglobin, the oxygen carrying pigment in our blood.

Fiber provides several benefits in the digestive system. It provides bulk and slows the emptying of the stomach which makes us feel full. It can bind unwanted substances like cholesterol or triglycerides and prevent us from reabsorbing them from our intestines, and it provides bulk for the bowel and helps to normalize movement of the large intestine. It has also been shown to reduce the incidence of bowel cancer.[31]

Also included in the category of nutritional supplements are the herbal substances which have been shown to have certain desirable actions in the body. These actions include thermogenesis or increase in metabolic rate, antioxidation, and chelation.

Thermogenics increase the metabolic rate. This causes more calories to be consumed than would normally be used over a given time period.

Part of the aging process involves the combination of our cellular structure with oxygen. This is the same process a piece of paper goes through when it burns, a nail goes through when it rusts, or a pile of garbage goes through when it decomposes. This process is called oxidation. In our bodies this process is caused by the availability of some types of molecules, called free radicals, for combination with oxygen. Antioxidants bind to these free radicals and prevent oxidation from occurring. It has been recognized by the medical community that antioxidants can slow, and in some cases, reverse the aging process. Antioxidants have also been acknowledged as being preventive for hardening of the arteries and some forms of cancer.

Chelation of minerals is a process of wrapping them in protein so that an efficient transport mechanism can be used for their absorption. This allows them to be absorbed into the body more readily. The absorption of minerals is usually by a cellular method called ionic pumping. This is an inefficient method of transportation, and, while it's fine as long as there is no deficit of a mineral, it's not efficient enough to build up stores once they've been used up.

I strongly recommend the use of nutritional supplements to my weight loss patients as a way to minimize the stresses of dieting and to compensate for the negative nutritional state produced by weight loss. This is especially important for patients under eighteen who need extra vitamins and minerals because of their active growth. Older people also have special needs because of depletion of stores and loss of efficiency of their metabolic processes.

# CHAPTER 12
# Informed Consent

When you talk with a doctor about a weight loss program, you have a right to have information about the benefits and risks so that you can make your own decision. Take the case of Jackie.

> Jackie is a pharmaceutical rep. She visits doctors offices every day, tells them about her company's medications, and encourages the doctors to consider using them in the course of his or her practice. The people chosen for this kind of job are very bright, pleasant, and usually fairly knowledgeable about their products. Jackie is twenty eight years old, 5'6" tall and weighs 138 pounds. She had a little girl two years

ago and wants to take off that last ten pounds. In the course of her job, one of the doctors she visited gave her a prescription for Redux®, and told her to take one a day. When she came to my office she asked me about the medication she was taking because she saw that I was actively offering a weight loss program.

I showed Jackie the prescribing information that comes with Redux® and explained the risks of Primary Pulmonary Hypertension. I also told her that, in my opinion, there was no way on the face of the earth to justify exposing her to those risks, especially without telling her about them first. She was horrified. Jackie doesn't take Redux® any more.

I guess the doctor thought he was doing her a favor. Some favor.

No one expects you to know as much about the medications that your doctor recommends as your doctor knows. We spend years learning about this stuff, and you have the right to expect that we understand the risks and consequences.

That does **not** mean that doctors have the right to choose whether you should be exposed to these risks. Our responsibility is to make recommendations based on our opinions and to clearly explain those risks to you. The final decision is yours. That's what informed consent is all about.

Informed consent also needs to involve both parents of the minor patient as well as anyone with a legal interest in that person.

Informed consent means that you have given your consent to your doctor for the recommended treatment *after* information has been provided to you. That information must be everything a reasonable person might need to know before making that decision. Informed consent is deemed to have been given when you have signed on the "dotted line" showing that you have had the opportunity to review the information and agree to the treatment.

The first element of informed consent is an honest disclosure of the effectiveness of the program. Based on Weintraub's research findings,[31] I use the 40% number to predict my patient's success with phen fen. Some people are disappointed when they compare the truth to what they've heard in the media, but I go on to point out that 40% is a lot better than less than 5% like the fad diets. When I don't have objective information on the effectiveness of a particular medication, I tell that to the patient as well.

The second element of informed consent is an honest disclosure of the risks associated with the appetite suppressants that you will be taking.

It is my opinion that adults who needs to lose 10% of their weight, and some adolescents who need to lose 20% of their weight, have enough medical need to justify the risks of appetite suppressants. It is your responsibility *once informed of the risks* to decide whether they are justifiable in your terms. The risk of Primary Pulmonary Hypertension is a perfect example of the kind of risks you need to consider. (See Appendix A under Redux®

for an explanation of Primary Pulmonary Hypertension). You have the right to be made aware of this risk before you are asked to decide whether to take these medications.

After explaining the increase in risk of Primary Pulmonary Hypertension (PPH) associated with the use of Pondimin® and Redux®, I offer my patients three choices.

1) The patient finds the risk acceptable and chooses not to limit the choice of appetite suppressants.

2) The patient chooses not to take either Pondimin® or Redux®.

3) The patient chooses to use the appetite suppressants not associated with the risk of PPH first and will consider taking the risk only if the other medications don't work.

I make sure to tell people that there are no wrong choices. The one that's right for you is the one you can be comfortable with while you're on the program. The only wrong choice is one that you don't get to make for yourself. Remember, your doctor does not have the right to make that decision for you.

In my experience, about 40% of people choose not to take either Pondimin® or Redux® once they are given the facts, even if it was their intention to take it when they first came to my office. This also applies to patients already taking either of these medications prescribed by another doctor.

If your doctor doesn't make you a part of the decision process then you should find one who will. Don't be afraid to ask questions. It's your life.

(A copy of my informed consent forms is included in Appendix B of this book.)

## CHAPTER 13

# Follow-Up

---

The last component of a well designed program, proper follow-up, is also one of the most important safety features.

At the beginning of your program, I recommend that you see your doctor every week for two weeks. If things are going well, you can then go every two weeks. Once you reach your weight-loss goals, follow-up could continue at one month, then two months later, and then every three months as long as you are taking your medication. Remember that this is not a temporary fix. These medications don't cure overweight, they just control it. You may need to be on appetite suppressants the rest of your life if you want to stay thin.

There are several areas that need to be checked at each follow-up visit.

### *Level of Hunger*

Assessing your level of hunger is an important ongoing issue. Until I, as your doctor, have done my job, that is effectively suppressed your hunger, neither you nor I have the right to expect you to follow a diet.

Sometimes it's difficult for you to know whether your hunger is adequately suppressed. After being on the program for awhile, some people tend to assume that they know what they're supposed to eat, and they go back to their old eating habits and stop losing weight. The only way to know whether failure to lose weight is caused by lack of compliance with the diet or by the reappearance of hunger is to use a clearly defined diet as a reference point. If hunger is the problem, you won't be able to follow the diet. If hunger is not the problem, you'll be able to resume your weight loss once you begin to follow the diet more carefully.

### *Amount of Weight Change*

It's important that you not lose weight too quickly or too slowly. Remember that the diet is designed to take off about two pounds per week.

If much less than two pounds is lost per week, the effectiveness of the medication has to be examined. If much more than two pounds are lost per week, the medication may be working too well and will be exposing you to the risks of malnutrition. In these cases, the dosage of the medication may need to be reduced.

The goal of the program is good health as well as weight control, not thinness at any cost.

## *Health Status*

Many of the appetite suppressants can cause elevations in blood pressure. Some people have pre-existing health problems which need to be watched carefully. Periodic re-evaluations of blood work or an electrocardiogram may be necessary to insure safety on the program. These types of issues have to be considered at each follow-up visit.

## *Medication Side Effects*

Almost everyone experiences some side effects when they start taking the medication. They range in severity from a dry mouth to inability to urinate and run the gamut of everything in between. The majority of these are mild and disappear after a week or two. However, if they are severe enough or persist long enough, it may be necessary to modify the dosage of the medication, or, occasionally, to stop it altogether. The effectiveness of a medication is not only measured by how well it works but by how tolerable it is for the patient to take.

It's up to you, not the doctor, to decide whether a side effect is tolerable. It is, however, important to try and put up with side effects for a short time to see whether they go away.

**Compliance**

In diet programs unassisted by appetite suppressants, you are expected to comply with the program, as well as the diet, *in spite of the fact that you are hungry.* In this program, compliance is an expectation that you will take the medication as prescribed and *try* to follow the diet whether or not you're hungry. As we've seen earlier in this chapter, the diet is a reference point for whether your hunger is well controlled, not for whether you are behaving well or badly.

## Hunger is the enemy, not your behavior.

# CHAPTER 14

# Giving It up

In our society we are taught that we are responsible for our own behaviors. This concept of responsibility is drilled into us from the time we are first able to think. I am a firm believer in this philosophy, because it makes us accountable for those behaviors *over which we have control*.

The difficulty with this philosophy is in understanding the difference between the areas over which we have control and those over which we do not. The serenity prayer says it best:

# Lord, grant me the serenity to *accept* the things I cannot change, the *courage* to change the things I can, and the *wisdom* to know the difference.

### *The Serenity to Accept*

We cannot change our genetic heritage. It makes us the beautiful people that we are, as well as all of the things about ourselves that drive us crazy, like our weight. It defines the machine — our body — that carries us around inside it, and, to some extent, it also defines the way our brains work.

Wellness includes the serenity to accept our individual identities and to love ourselves because of, and in spite of, who we are. Any process, or understanding, or theory, that fails to allow us to do this is *morally wrong*.

Just as we accept that it is wrong to judge a person by the color of his or her skin, or by the way that he or she worships, so we should accept that it is morally wrong for us, or anyone else, to judge who we are by our weight. This is not a permissive attitude. It is a recognition that our natural weight is one of the basic aspects of our identity.

### *The Courage to Change*

Overweight people have shown great courage in the face of adversity for a very long time — courage against tremendous prejudice and courage in our attempts to change something over which we had no control.

Dieting, which has been the only means we've been offered to deal with overweight, has given us an impossible task — to overcome our natural genetic identities by the use of will power alone or suffer the consequences of overweight.

We need to use our courage, not to change our natures, but to change the way we think about our weight. That courage should be used to stop blaming ourselves for our lack of success with traditional diets. We also need the courage to reject the guilt and blame placed on us by ignorant people and begin to demand the same respectful treatment from the medical community that is given for any chronic unwellness.

### *The Wisdom to Know the Difference*

We need the wisdom to *give it up* — in the sense of releasing the self-blame about our natural weight — to a higher power, one which I have called Mother Nature but which you may call by another name. Part of the process of *giving it up* is gaining the wisdom to understand that we do not have voluntary control over our weight and acknowledging that the means to that control must come from outside ourselves.

Use this wisdom to seek that help through a doctor who will work with you over the long-term to the best of his or her ability, without any guarantees, and without any blame.

The wisdom to know the difference brings with it the ability to give up the blame, guilt, fault, and fear. With this understanding comes the greatest reward of all, the freedom to accept yourself as a good person.

**GOOD HEALTH.**

# APPENDIX A

# The Appetite Suppressants

This appendix describes the effective appetite suppressants currently available in this country. **This information is not comprehensive. Many possible side effects, complications, contraindications, and precautions are not included in this book. This information is intended to provide you with basic information about the appetite suppressants so that you can discuss them with your doctor.**

One common characteristic of all the appetite suppressants is that they interfere with the hunger signals produced by the hypothalamus in one way or another. Some make serotonin more available in the brain like some antidepressants such as Prozac do. Some increase the availability of norepinephrine, another neurotransmitter, while others have mechanisms of action that are poorly understood. Regardless of their mechanism, they have all been shown to be effective for appetite suppression.

Because of their neurotransmitter action on serotonin and norepinephrine, these medications should not be stopped suddenly because of the risk of acute depression. This is not an issue of addiction. There are many other types of medications that shouldn't be suddenly stopped such as propranalol, anticonvulsants, and antidepressants, to name a few.

If you need to stop taking these medications, do so slowly over a period of weeks. Always consult with your doctor first. It is also important that you report to your doctor any symptoms you experience while taking appetite suppressants, even if you think the problems are unrelated to the medication.

Over-the-counter appetite suppressants will be discussed in the next section, followed by the prescription medications.

### *Over-the-Counter Appetite Suppressants*

## **Phenylpropanolamine HCL, (PPA); Brand Names: Acutrim® and Dexatrim® (slow-release)**

This medication is available in two forms. The quick release form must be taken several times a day. The slow-release form, sold as Dexatrim® and Acutrim®, can be taken once a day. Many of the patients I see have already tried Acutrim® or Dexatrim® and are very skeptical when I suggest the use of PPA. Only after I explain the difference in effectiveness between the long-acting and short-acting forms are they willing to try PPA again.

I place my patients who are taking the short acting form of PPA on the same type of program as my patients who are on prescription appetite suppressants. Although not everyone responds to PPA, it is generally very effective, even if you need to lose a hundred pounds.

Although this is a non-prescription medication, it should only be taken in a properly designed weight loss program, not on your own! Imagine going into a pharmacy, sticking your arm in a blood pressure monitor and finding out you've got high blood pressure. You go to the blood pressure pill section and choose the prettiest package, leave the store, and take a pill every day. What if there is a reversible reason for your elevated blood pressure? How do you know if the medication you've chosen is safe for you? What do you do about any side effects?

Taking PPA without a well-designed program monitored by a doctor is dangerous, and it reduces your chances for long-term success on the one medication that may be right for you. It's the only medication I feel is safe enough for those who need to lose less than 10% of their body weight. However, I also use it for my more overweight patients.

Remember, it's not about the medications. It's about suppressing the appetite safely and effectively.

## *Effectiveness*

In some studies, the quick-release form of phenylpropanolamine has been shown to be twice as effective in suppressing the appetite as the slow-release form.[32] In many cases, it has been shown to be *just as effective as the prescription medications!*[33] The quick release form of PPA is not generally available in most pharmacies, but it can usually be ordered.

## *Side Effects*

PPA has some of the same potential stimulant side effects as the prescribed appetite suppressants. It is generally considered to be safer than the prescription medications, with less severe side effects. Potential side effects of PPA include:

- Fast heart rate
- Insomnia
- Agitation
- Dry mouth
- Diarrhea

## *Dosage*

The dosage of PPA non-slow release is 25 mg. one hour before each meal.

# Ephedrine

This over-the-counter medication has been used in various forms as a decongestant and stimulant for many years. Studies done in the last few years have shown ephedrine to be effective in promoting weight loss especially when combined with caffeine[34].

However, ephedrine has not been approved for use in weight loss in the United States because of concerns about its stimulant nature, especially on the cardiovascular system. The side effects of ephedrine are directly related to dosage, and it is easy to take too much in an effort to lose weight. Ephedrine can be life-threatening at high dosage.

Because of the potential for very serious side effects and because the proper formulations for weight loss are not available, I do not recommend its use for weight loss at this time. There may be a role for ephedrine in a properly supervised program in the future but only after research provides us with better information about its effectiveness and safety.

## *Prescription Appetite Suppressants*

There are seven different prescription appetite suppressants available. They fall into two basic categories. The first, and most common category, is the sympathomimetic amines. All this very impressive name means is that they mimic the effect of adrenaline in the body, and, therefore, are stimulant in nature. All of the appetite suppressants, with the exception of fenfluramine and dexfenfluramine, fall into this group. These make up the second category, the antihistiminics which tend to have sedative side effects.

Only some of the more common brand names for the medications will be listed in this section. The newest medication available, Redux® will be listed first, followed by the phen fen combination and the remaining choices.

## **Dexfenfluramine**, Brand Name: **Redux®**

Dexfenfluramine (Redux®) is the newest appetite suppressant approved by the FDA. However, it has been available in Europe for many years. The medical community there has recognized it as an effective appetite suppressant which doesn't cause addiction. France has restricted its use to people who are at least 30% over their ideal weight because of the associated side effect of Primary Pulmonary Hypertension.

Primary Pulmonary Hypertension (PPH) has been associated with the use of dexfenfluramine (Redux®) and dl fenfluramine (Pondimin®), the second half of phen fen.[35] PPH is a rare but devastating disease which results from the development of resistance to blood flow through the lungs. It can result in the need for a heart lung transplant and causes death in about 55% of those affected. The risk of PPH in the general population is two cases per million people. If you factor in the use of phenfluramine and dexfenfluramine, this number jumps to up to forty-six per million. This is a twenty-three-fold increase in risk (forty-four extra cases) per million. While this is still a relatively small risk, those extra forty-four people will still wish they'd never heard of these medications. About twenty-three of them will eventually die. The risk is increased as the length of time on the medication and the dosage are increased.

The importance of Redux® in its approval by the FDA is *in spite* of its association with PPH. This represents a shift in the attitude of the regulatory and medical communities to a view that overweight is a serious health risk and that some risk is acceptable in the treatment of overweight.

Dexfenfluramine is similar in structure to dl fenfluramine. They are both antihistaminic appetite suppressants and are about equally effective in producing weight loss. However, some report reduced side effects with dexfenfluramine.

In my opinion, the research on Redux® does not indicate any obvious benefit over dl fenfluramine. I prescribe it, but not necessarily as first choice, because the studies by Weintraub showed phen fen to be effective for a longer period than dexfenfluramine. However, it was a longer study. I want to see head-to-head comparisons before I pass final judgment on Redux®.

### *Effectiveness*

The effectiveness of Redux® is reported as a weight loss of at least 10% of starting weight after a period of one year by 40% of people taking it.[36]

### *Side Effects*

Because Redux® is an antihistiminic, it tends to have sedative side effects. The most common side effects include:

- Tiredness
- Diarrhea

- Dry mouth
- Drowsiness

These symptoms are usually mild and resolve soon after starting the medication.

## *Dosage*

The dosage of dexfenfluramine is 15 mg. in the morning and evening.

## **dl Fenfluramine ("fen"), Brand Name: Pondimin®**

This medication is one half of the phen fen combination which started the rebirth of appetite suppressant use in this country. It been used alone for many years and in combination with phentermine since about 1992. The combination of phen fen is felt to reduce the side effects of both medications and increase their lengths of action.

## *Effectiveness*

The effectiveness of dl fenfluramine alone has not been adequately studied. In combination with phentermine, it has been shown to cause more than 10% weight loss in up to 40% of people who took it for about three years.[39]

## *Side Effects*

As the only other antihistaminic appetite suppressant, its side effects are generally sedating. They are nicely offset by the stimulant side effects of phentermine. Like Redux®, this medication has also been associated with

Primary Pulmonary Hypertension.[38] The most common side effects include:

- Dry mouth
- Nausea
- Diarrhea
- Drowsiness or lethargy
- Light-headedness

These symptoms often go away after a few days use.

### *Dosage*

The dosage of fenfluramine is 20 mg. two or three times a day, about one hour before meals. Weintraub suggests that fenfluramine may be effective in lesser dosages when combined with phentermine. My clinical experience has not always shown this to be true. I have patients who take fenfluramine once, twice, and three times a day. Whatever dosage is effective is the dosage that should be used.

### **Phentermine Resin ("phen"), Brand Name: Ionamin®, and Phentermine HCl, Brand Names: Adipex P® or Fastin®**

Phentermine resin (Ionamin®), the other half of the phen fen combination, stays in the bloodstream longer and has a slower onset of action than phentermine HCl. This may lessen the side effects of the medication in some people. I recommend the use of phentermine resin rather than phentermine HCL because it was the form used in the Weintraub study. Phentermine has been used alone since the seventies and in combination with fenfluramine since about 1992.

## Effectiveness

The effectiveness of phentermine alone has not been adequately studied. In combination with dl fenfluramine, it has been shown to cause more than 10% weight loss in up to 40% of people who took it for about three years.[39]

## Side Effects

Phentermine is a sympathomimetic amine and stimulant in nature. The side effects of phentermine include:

- Insomnia
- Nervousness
- Headache

## Dosage

The dosage of Ionamin® is 15 or 30 mg. once in the morning. Adipex-P® is taken in doses of 37.5 mg. before breakfast. Fastin® is taken in doses of 30 mg. before breakfast.

# Benzphetamine HCL, Brand Name: Didrex®

This is the most amphetamine-like of the appetite suppressants available in this country. It is a sympathomimetic amine and has stimulant types of side effects. One of the problems with taking this medication is that urine drug testing will not distinguish this medication from the illegal amphetamines. This should be kept in mind by patients who might be subject to drug testing.

Appendix A

## *Effectiveness*

Benzphetamine HCL has been shown to be an effective appetite suppressant.

## *Side Effects*

- Dry mouth
- Insomnia
- Nervousness

## *Dosage*

The dosage of benzphetamine HCL is up to 50 mg. three times a day.

## **Diethylpropion HCL**, Brand Name: **Tenuate**®, **Tenuate Dosespan**®

Diethylpropion has been used effectively since the seventies. This medication is usually well tolerated and very effective for some people. Better studies on this medication are needed and its use should increase as its effectiveness and safety are better known.

## *Effectiveness*

Diethylpropion has been shown to be an effective appetite suppressant.

## *Side Effects*

This medication is one of the sympathomemetic amines and is stimulant in nature. The most common side effects include:

- Insomnia
- Nervousness
- Dry mouth

## Dosage

The dosage of diethylpropion HCL is either 25 mg. one hour before each meal. In the case of the long-acting form, 75 mg. is taken once in the morning.

## **Mazindol**, Brand Name: **Sanorex**®

This medication may have a different mechanism of action than the others. It would be interesting to see some studies on a combination of this medication with one of the others. My clinical experience has shown that when it works, it's great. But it may be effective for a smaller proportion of people than some of the other appetite suppressants.

### *Effectiveness*

Mazindol is an effective appetite suppressant.

### *Side Effects*

This medication is also a sympathomemetic amine and stimulant in nature. The most common side effects of mazindol are:

- Dry mouth
- Constipation
- Abdominal discomfort
- Nausea

- Sleep disturbance
- Dizziness

Most people have some side effects with mazindol, but these tend to be mild and go away after a few days to a few weeks.

### *Dosage*

The dosage of mazindol is 1 mg. up to three times a day.

### **Phendimetrazine Tartrate; Brand Names: Bontril® (slow-release) or Prelu-2® (time-release).**

My experience with this medication has been very positive. Many of my patients who have not had good appetite suppression with other medications have found phendimetrazine to be very effective. I start with the short-acting form and, if it works, then try the longer acting form. The two forms do not always work equally well in any individual patient.

### *Effectiveness*

Phendimetrazine tartrate is an effective appetite suppressant.

### *Side Effects*

This medication is a sympathomimetic amine. The side effects of include:

- Dry mouth
- Nausea

- Constipation
- Dizziness

These symptoms usually resolve within a short time of use.

## *Dosage*

The dosage of phendimetrazine tartrate is 35 mg. three times a day, or one 105 mg. slow release tablet before breakfast.

## **New Medications**

### **Sibutramine**, Brand Name: **Meridia**®

Research is currently being conducted on a new appetite suppressant known generically as sibutramine[40] and which will be marketed as Meridia®. Studies have shown this medication to be effective. However, the dosage necessary for this effectiveness have been associated with the side effects of insomnia, irritability, impatience, and excitation.

### **Orlistat**, Brand Name: **Xenical**®

Another medication under study for weight loss is orlistat. The brand name will be Xenical®. This medication blocks the effect of lipase, an enzyme necessary for the breakdown of fat in the intestine. Studies have shown it to be effective in reducing fat absorption which causes weight loss.[41] The two problems associated with orlistat have been the reduction of absorption of the fat soluble vitamins A, D, E, and K and the gastrointestinal problems associated with the mal-absorption of fat, such as flatulence, intestinal cramping, and bloating.

# APPENDIX B

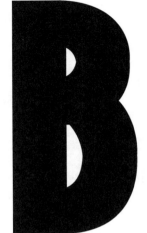

# Informed Consent Forms

These forms have been written by the author and are not in any way authoritative. They do not represent any standard but that used by the author in the course of his practice.

## The General Risks Of Weight Loss

Change of any type is always associated with risk. Weight loss is no exception. Some of the risks you face are associated with the loss of weight itself and some of the risks are specific to the particular program you follow.

First, let's look at the general risks of weight loss.

1) Gall bladder disease
   The gall bladder concentrates bile. When less bile is produced during weight loss the gall bladder may form stones. This could require surgery to treat, and surgery is risky.

2) Loss of lean body mass
   Some loss of lean body mass is expected, such as loss of water. Loss of bone or muscle can be a serious side effect of some programs. While this program is specifically designed to prevent this from happening, the risk of bone or muscle mass loss still exists.

3) Loss of hair
   This is more common in programs which reduce calories dramatically. However any stress such as caloric restriction can cause hair loss.

4) Change in bowel habits
   Diarrhea or constipation can occur with change in diet. These are usually temporary and can be managed within your program.

5) Indigestion or heartburn
   You may not "use up" all of the acid in your stomach when you eat less. It may be necessary to neutralize the acid or reduce its production at the start of the program.

6) Change in menstrual cycle
   Hormones are stored in fat. As the level of fat in your body changes it may affect the hormonal cycles of your body. Your periods could become irregular.

7) Coldness
Some people feel cold when they lose their "insulation."

# Risks Specific To This Program

These are the risks associated with the program your doctor has designed for you. These risks will depend partly on the appetite suppressants you are prescribed. Those chosen for you are circled.

1) Risks associated with phentermine (Ionamin®)
These can include, but are not limited to, increased blood pressure, insomnia, tremor, headache, dry mouth (common), diarrhea, constipation, hives, and changes in sex drive. A reprint of the *Physician's Desk Reference* section on phentermine is available at your request.

2) Risks associated with fenfluramine (Pondimin®)
These can include, but are not limited to, drowsiness, dry mouth, diarrhea, confusion, headache, fatigue, nausea, Urinary frequency, increased or decreased blood pressure. A reprint of the *Physician's Desk Reference* section on fenfluramine is available at your request.

3) Risks associated with dexfenfluramine (Redux®)
These can include, but are not limited to, tiredness, diarrhea, dry mouth, and drowsiness. A reprint of the manufacturer's package insert on Redux® is available at your request.

NOTE: Primary Pulmonary Hypertension has been seen as a side effect of fenfluramine (Pondimin®) and dexfenfluramine (Redux®). This is an unpredictable complication, which is fatal in 55% of cases, or which could result in the need of a heart-lung transplant. This can occur long after the medication is stopped. While this is a rare complication, it is very serious. Each person should consider whether he or she is willing to take this risk. Shortness of breath should be immediately reported to your doctor. The incidence of Primary Pulmonary Hypertension is two cases per million people in the general population. With the use of either fenfluramine or dexfenfluramine this incidence rises to up to forty-six cases per million people, a twenty-three-fold increase in risk.

It is important that you make your own decision as to whether you are willing to take either Pondimin® or Redux® in the face of this risk. There are three decisions available for you to make. **There are no wrong decisions!** Please indicate which one you decide by circling your choice.

    A) I do not wish to be exposed to the risk of Primary Pulmonary Hypertension, and do not wish to take either Pondimin® or Redux®.

    B) I understand the risk of Primary Pulmonary Hypertension associated with taking either Pondimin® or Redux®, and I have decided to take that risk.

    C) I do not wish to take the risk of Primary Pulmonary Hypertension if I can reach my weight loss goals without using either Pondimin® or Redux®, but I may be willing to reconsider taking those risks if the other medications do not work.

Appendix B

4) <u>Risks associated with phendimetrazine tartrate</u>
These can include, but are not limited to, dry mouth, nausea, diarrhea, dizziness. A reprint of *The Physician's Desk Reference* section on phendimetrazine tartrate is available at your request.

5) <u>Risks associated with mazindol</u>
These can include, but are not limited to, dry mouth, constipation, abdominal discomfort, nausea, sleep disturbance, dizziness. Mazindol should not be taken by people who have a history of seizures. A reprint of *The Physician's Desk Reference* section on mazindol is available at your request.

6) <u>Risks associated with diethylpropion (Tenuate®)</u>
These can include but are not limited to, insomnia, dry mouth, nervousness. A reprint of *The Physician's Desk Reference* section on diethylpropion is available at your request.

7) <u>Risks associated with benzphetamine HCL (Didrex®)</u>
These can include, but are not limited to, insomnia, dry mouth, and nervousness. A reprint of *The Physician's Desk Reference* section on benzphetamine HCL is available at your request.

8) <u>Risks of stopping medication improperly</u>
These medications must be discontinued under a doctor's supervision. If you decide to discontinue the use of either or both of these medications severe depression may occur unless this is done slowly. Your doctor will respect your wishes and prescribe a program of gradual withdrawal. This is not an addictive problem but one based on the neurochemical effects of the medications.

9) <u>Risks associated with length of use</u>
With the exception of Redux® all of the appetite suppressants have been approved by the FDA for use of "a few weeks" duration. This is contrary to your doctors intention. Your doctor intends to prescribe these medications for you for an indefinite time.

10) <u>Risks associated with nutritional supplements</u>
The nutritional products recommended by your doctor are not subject to the same level of oversight as prescription medications with regard to safety and effectiveness. It is possible that individual responses could occur to some of the ingredients. A complete list of these ingredients is available for your inspection.


I have read and understood "The Risks of Weight Loss." I have decided to participate in the program.

Patient's name    _____

Patient's signature_____

# APPENDIX C

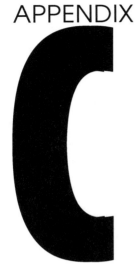

# References

1. M. Weintraub, "Long Term Weight Control Study: Conclusions," *Clinical Pharmacology and Therapeutics (U.S.)* 51(5) (May 1992): 642-46.
2. R. J. Kuczmarski et al., "Increasing Prevalence of Overweight among US Adults. The National Health and Nutrition Examination Surveys, 1960 to 1991," *Journal of the American Medical Association (U.S.)* 272(3) (July 20, 1994): 205-11.
3. P. Sorlie et al., "Body Build and Mortality. The Framingham Study.," *Journal of the American Medical Association (U.S.)* 243(18) (May 1980): 1828-831.
4. D. Blair et al., "Evidence of an Increased Risk for Hypertension with Centrally Located Body Fat and

the Effect of Race and Sex on this Risk," *American Journal of Epidemiology (U.S.)* 119(4) (Apr 1984): 526-40.
5. S. Popkess-Vawter, "Reducing Cardiac Risk Factors in the Obese Patient," *Nursing Clinics of North America (U.S.)* 17(2) (June 1982): 233-44.
6. R. Shinton et al., "Body Fat and Stroke: Unmasking the Hazards of Overweight and Obesity," *Journal of Epidemiology and Community Health (England)* 49(3) (June 1995): 259-64.
7. L. E. Tucker et al., "Prevalence of Gallstones in Obese Caucasian American Women," *International Journal of Obesity (England)* 6(3) (1982): 247-51.
8. H. Maegawa et al., "Obesity as a Risk Factor for Developing Non-Insulin Dependent Diabetes Melitus—Obesity and Insulin Resistance," *Nippon Naibunpi Gakkai Zasshi (Japan)* 71(2) (March 20, 1995): 97-104.
9. K. Hakala et al., "Effect of Weight Loss and Body Position on Pulmonary Function and Gas Exchange Abnormalities in Morbid Obesity," *International Journal of Obesity Related Metabolic Disorders (England)* 19(5) (May 1995): 343-46.
10. B. T. Emmesson, "The Management of Gout," *New England Journal of Medicine (U.S.)* 334(7) (February 15, 1996): 445-51.
11. F. de Waard et al., "Relationship of Weight to the Promotion of Breast Cancer after Menopause," *Nutrition and Cancer (U.S.)* 2(4) (1981): 237-40.
12. A. S. Vishnevskii et al., "Multifactorial Analysis of the Effect of Metabolic and Endocrine Factors on Cellular Immunity in Patients with Cancer of the Uterine Body," *Akush Ginekol (Mosk) (USSR)* (2) (1990): 38-42.
13. C. La Vecchia et al., "Oestrogens and Obesity as Risk Factors for the Endometrial Cancer in Italy," *International Journal of Epidemiology (England)* 11(2) (June

1982)": 120-26.
14. D. A. Snowon et al., "Diet, Obesity, and Risk of Fatal Prostate Cancer," *American Journal of Epidemiology (U.S.)*, 120(2) (August 1984): 244-45.
15. E. Giovannucci et al., "Physical Activity, Obesity, and Risk for Colon Cancer and Adenoma in Men," *Annals of Internal Medicine (U.S.)* 122(5) (March 1, 1995,): 327-34.
16. L. N. Kolonel et al., "Epidemiology of Testicular Cancer in the Pacific Basin," *National Cancer Institute Monograph (U.S.)* 62 (1982): 157-60.
17. P. S. Choban et al., "Increased Incidence of Nosocomial Infections in Obese Surgical Patients," *American Surgeon (U.S.)* 61(11) (November 1995): 1001-05.
18. S. R. Johnson et al., "Maternal Obesity and Pregnancy," *Surgical Gynecological Obstet rics (U.S.)* 164(5) (May 1987): 431-37.
19. Ibid., 2.
20. W. S. Browner et al., "What if Americans Ate Less Fat? A Quantitative Estimate of the Effect on Mortality," *Journal of the American Medical Association (U.S)* 265(24) (June 26, 1991): 3285-91.
21. L. M. Smith-Schneider et al., "Dietary Fat Reduction Strategies," *Journal of the American Dietetic Association (U.S.)* 92(1) (January 1992): 34-38.
22. B. J. Rolls et al., "Satiety After Preloads with Different Amounts of Fat and Carbohydrate: Implications for Obesity," *American Journal of Clinical Nutrition (U.S.)* 60(4) (October 1994): 476-87.
23. R. P. Blank et al., "Calcium Metabolism and Osteoporotic Ridge Resorption: A Protein Connection," *Journal of Prosthetic Dentistry (U.S.)* 58(5) (November 1987): 590-95.
24. G. M. Janssen et al., "Food Intake and Body Composition in Novice Athletes during a Training Period to

Run a Maratho," *International Journal of Sports Medicine (U.S.)* No. 10 (1989) Sup 1: 17-21.
25. G. W. Gleim, "Exercise is not an Effective Weight Loss Modality in Women," *Journal of the American College of Nutrition (U.S.)* 12(4) (August 12, 1993): 363-67.
26. S. Shinkai et al., "Effects of 12 Weeks of Aerobic Exercise Plus Dietary Restriction on Body Composition, Resting Energy Expenditure and Aerobic Fitness in Mildly Obese Middle-aged Women," *European Journal of Applied Physiology (Germany)* 68(3) (1994): 258-65.
27. K. D. Brownell et al., "Changes in Plasma Lipid and Lipoprotein Levels in Men and Women After a Program of Moderate Exercise," *Circulation (U.S.)* 65(3) ( March 1982): 477-84.
28. H. Yamasaki et al., "Effects of Weight Training on Muscle Strength and Exercise Capacity in Patients after Myocardial Infarction," *Journal of Cardiology (Japan)* 26(6) (December): 341-47.
29. B. P. Abernathy et al., "Healthy Body Weights: An Alternative Perspective," *American Journal of Clinical Nutrition (U.S.)*, 63 (March 1996) sup 3: 448s-451s.
30. Ibid., 1.
31. J. H. Weisburger et al., "Protective Mechanisms of Dietary Fibers in Nutritional Carcinogenesis," *Basic Life Science (U.S.)* 61 (1993): 45-63,
32. Y. X. Shen et al., "Comparison of Multiple Dosage Bioavailability Between Phenylpropanolamine Controlled Release Suspension and Conventional Tablet in Healthy Volunteers," *Yao Hsueh Hsueh Pao (China)* 30(2) (1995): 157-60.
33. T. Silverstone, "Appetite Suppressants. A Review," *Drugs (New Zealand)* 43(6) (Jun 1992): 820-36.
34. A. Astrup et al., "The Effect and Safety of an Ephedrin/ Caffeine Compound Compared to Ephedrin, Caffeine

and Placebo in Obese Subjects on an Energy Restricted Diet. A Double Blind Trial," *International Journal of Obesity Related Metabolic Disorders (England)* 16(4) (April 1992): 269-77.
35. S. H. Thomas et al., "Appetite Suppressants and Primary Pulmonary Hypertension in the United Kingdom," *British Heart Journal (England)* (December 1995), 74(6): 660-3.
36. Manufacturer's product insert.
37. Ibid., 1.
38. Ibid., 35.
39. Ibid., 1.
40. M. Weintraub et al., "Sibutramine in Weight Control: A Dose Ranging, Efficacy Study," *Clinical and Pharmacological Therapeutics (U.S.)* (September 1991) 50(3): 330-7
41. M. L. Brent et al., "Orlistat (Ro 18-0647), A Lipase Inhibitor, in the Treatment of Human Obesity: A Multiple Dose Study," *International Journal of Obesity and Related Metabolic Disorders (England)*, 19(4) (April 1995): 221-26.